Energy Stability

How the Body Regulates Fuel, Fatigue, Recovery, and Daily Function

Nathan Reed

PERENNIAL PUBLISHING

Published by Perennial Publishing

Paperback ISBN: 978-1-971996-51-6
Hardcover ISBN: 978-1-971996-52-3
E-book ISBN: 978-1-971996-53-0

Contents

Energy as Functional Output

Energy is familiar because it is felt before it is analyzed. It arrives as readiness, fatigue, heaviness, clarity, fog, alertness, resistance, motion, urgency, or inconsistency. A person does not first encounter energy as a metabolic diagram. Energy appears in the body as the ability to begin, continue, shift attention, move through ordinary demand, tolerate effort, recover from strain, or feel the loss of those capacities.

Because energy is felt directly, it often appears obvious. Fatigue seems to explain itself because it is immediate. Alertness seems to explain itself because it changes behavior before it is questioned. Fog, heaviness, and crashes are not abstract ideas; they are experienced as changes in usable function. The signal arrives first. Interpretation follows.

That immediacy is useful, but it is also misleading. A feeling can be real without being complete. Low energy may be present before the system that produced it is understood. A crash may be felt suddenly even if the conditions that built it were developing earlier. A strong morning may feel like stability even if the pattern later becomes volatile. Energy is immediate, but immediacy does not make it self-explanatory.

This is why energy is one of the most commonly misread metabolic experiences. It is close enough to daily life that it seems simple, yet it is produced by many interacting layers. The body does not generate energy as a single isolated feeling. It produces usable function through fuel access, conversion, circulation, signaling, recovery, stress response, appetite, glucose movement, insulin coordination, electrolyte and fluid balance, load, and capacity.

Energy is often interpreted through the nearest visible explanation. When energy is low, the explanation may become lack of effort. When energy is high, it may be interpreted as motivation or strength. When fatigue appears, sleep may be treated as the only cause. When a crash follows a meal, food may become the entire explanation. When fog appears, stimulation may become the assumed missing piece. When energy changes unpredictably, inconsistency may be treated as personality.

Each of these interpretations can contain partial truth. Sleep matters. Food matters. Stimulation can change alertness. Effort and behavior are part of daily function. But partial explanations become distorted when they are treated as complete mechanisms. The nearest visible explanation is not always the whole system.

A person may sleep for a similar duration on two nights and feel different the next day because sleep quality, stress load, prior demand, glucose handling, appetite pressure, and recovery state changed. A meal may feel stabilizing in one context and heavy in another because the system receiving the meal is different. A period of alertness may come from restoration, but it may also come from stress activation or compensation. A crash may involve glucose movement, but it may also involve transition strain, poor recovery, accumulated load, or compensatory output reaching a limit.

Energy should not be reduced to motivation, discipline, or personality. High energy is not proof of virtue. Fatigue is not proof of weakness. Inconsistency is not automatically lack of seriousness. Alertness is not automatically motivation. A crash is not a personal failure. These states may shape behavior, but they should not be judged before they are understood.

This does not remove behavior from the picture. It removes moral reduction. Behavior occurs inside a system of constraints, signals, recovery state, and demand. The purpose of this book is not to excuse or blame. It is to explain. Energy patterns should be interpreted as system outputs before they are judged as personal traits.

Energy is also not sleep alone or food alone. Sleep is one of the major restoration layers beneath daily energy, but sleep does not explain every energy pattern by itself. Food enters the system as material, but intake alone does not determine usable energy. Calories may be present without smooth fuel access. Stored energy may exist without being readily available. Glucose may move visibly without explaining the entire energy state. Stimulation may raise alertness without creating durable capacity.

Energy emerges from coordination across systems. Fuel must become accessible. Accessible fuel must be converted into usable work. Fuel-state transitions must be tolerated. Glucose movement must be coordinated. Insulin must route energy across use, storage, circulation, and access. Appetite must translate internal state into behavioral pressure. Sleep must restore capacity. Stress must be absorbed without excessive cost. Electrolyte and fluid balance must support signal transmission, circulation, nerve activity, and muscle function. Load must remain within available capacity often enough for continuity to hold.

Energy, in this frame, is functional output. It is how the system's internal state becomes daily function. It appears as movement, attention, clarity, physical ease, tolerance, steadiness, recovery, and the ability to continue across ordinary demand. It includes physical function and cognitive continuity. It is not simply whether the body contains fuel. It is whether internal conditions can be translated into usable output.

A fuel gauge is too simple a model. A full fuel tank does not explain whether fuel can be accessed, routed, converted, and expressed. A high reading at one moment does not explain whether output will remain stable later. Energy is not one stored substance waiting to be spent. It is a regulated expression of many systems operating together.

This is why energy stability cannot be defined by intensity. A high-energy window may feel impressive, but it does not prove stability. A burst of alertness, urgency, stimulation, or momentum can produce output for a period while the underlying pattern remains fragile. If that output is followed by collapse, prolonged recovery, appetite disruption, irritability, fog, or baseline drift, the peak did not represent durable stability.

Energy stability is continuity, not intensity.

Continuity does not mean feeling elevated all day. It does not mean eliminating every dip. It does not require flatness, constant alertness, or a perfect line of output. Living systems move. Energy rises and falls with time of day, meals, sleep state, stress, activity, recovery, and demand. Stable energy allows rhythm.

Stable energy means usable output remains available across ordinary demand without excessive peaks, crashes, drift, or compensatory strain. It means variation is recoverable. It means lower-output periods do not repeatedly become collapses. It means output can soften without becoming unstable. It means the system can move without losing coherence.

Energy continuity is more important than energy intensity because continuity reveals whether the system can sustain function across time. Intensity shows what the system can produce briefly. Continuity shows whether that output can hold, recover, and remain proportionate. A moderate pattern that continues may represent greater stability than a high peak followed by sharp decline.

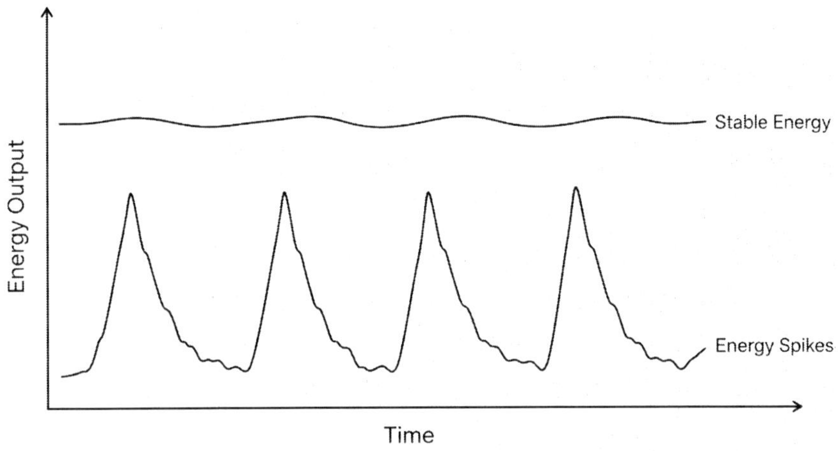

[Figure 1 — Energy Continuity vs Energy Peaks]

The central mechanism of this book is the Energy Continuity Mechanism. The Energy Continuity Mechanism explains how energy stability depends on the body's ability to sustain functional output across time without excessive peaks, crashes, drift, or compensatory strain.

This mechanism reframes energy from a peak state to a continuity pattern. It explains why high energy alone is not stability. It explains why fatigue, crashes, fog, heaviness, and inconsistency must be interpreted across time rather than judged as isolated moments. It also explains why energy can feel unstable even when one visible input appears unchanged.

A crash may be the delayed result of earlier instability. Drift may occur when baseline energy gradually lowers until reduced function feels normal. Compensation may preserve output temporarily while increasing future strain. Appetite may misalign with energy need. Glucose may influence perceived availability without explaining the whole system. Sleep may alter next-day capacity. Stress may raise alertness while increasing cost. Electrolyte and fluid balance may affect physical ease and fatigue perception. Load may exceed capacity even when each individual demand seems ordinary.

The Energy Continuity Mechanism gives these patterns a common frame. Energy is not interpreted by asking only whether it is high or low. It is interpreted by asking whether usable function holds across time, whether variation is recoverable, whether output depends on compensation, whether baseline is drifting, and whether load repeatedly exceeds capacity.

This book is not a productivity system. It is not a stimulant strategy. It is not a peak-performance manual. It is not a program for maximizing energy. It does not turn energy into another target to force upward. It does not offer protocols, routines, or promises of constant elevation.

The purpose of this book is to explain energy stability. It examines the system beneath energy: fuel availability, energy conversion, fuel-state transitions, glucose patterns, insulin signaling, appetite signals, sleep state, stress load, electrolyte and fluid balance, recovery, pattern recognition, load, and capacity. Each layer helps explain why energy holds, fluctuates, crashes, drifts, or requires compensation.

This boundary matters because energy is often pulled into performance language. It becomes something to increase, protect, chase, or measure against an idealized state. But energy stability is not about becoming constantly elevated. It is about understanding how the body sustains usable output under real conditions.

The book begins by separating output continuity from peak output. Chapter 1 introduces the Output Continuity Mechanism, which explains why energy should not be judged by isolated high-energy moments. A brief period of alertness may be useful, but usefulness is not the same as stability. A peak may show what the system can produce briefly; it does not show what the system can sustain.

The first step is therefore to define energy stability as continuity across time. Before crashes, drift, compensation, glucose, insulin, appetite, sleep, stress, electrolytes, load, and capacity can be understood, the central distinction must be clear: stable energy is not the highest point the system can reach. It is the ability of usable function to continue without repeated disruption.

Output Continuity Mechanism

Energy is often interpreted through its most noticeable moments. A period of sharp alertness, a sudden rise in motivation, a stretch of productive output, or a window in which effort feels unusually easy tends to stand out against the background of an otherwise ordinary day. These moments draw attention because they contrast with baseline experience. They feel distinct, elevated, and temporarily unbounded. Because they are so visible, they are often taken as evidence that the underlying system is functioning well.

This interpretation relies on a narrow slice of the system's behavior. It assumes that the most intense expression of energy reflects the system as a whole. A brief period of high output becomes a proxy for stability. If energy can rise to a noticeable level, it is assumed to be sufficient. If it feels strong at any point, it is interpreted as working. The rest of the day, including what precedes and follows that moment, is treated as secondary or unrelated.

This is a misreading of what energy represents.

A moment of elevated output does not describe the system's behavior across time. It captures a peak, not a pattern. It shows what the system can produce under a specific set of conditions, but it does not show whether that production can be sustained, repeated, or integrated into ongoing function without disruption. It does not show how the system transitions into that state or how it recovers from it. It does not reveal whether the output is supported by stable coordination or whether it is produced through temporary compensation.

The distinction between peak output and stable output begins here. Peak output is a momentary measurement. It answers a narrow question: how high did energy rise at a given point in time? It is defined by intensity. It captures the upper range of what the system can express, but it does so without context. It does not account for duration, continuity, or recovery. It is a snapshot, not a sequence.

Stable output operates under a different frame. It is not concerned with how high energy rises in isolated moments. It is concerned with whether usable function can continue across time without repeated interruption. It asks a different question: did function hold across time? This question shifts attention away from intensity and toward continuity. It requires observing how energy behaves before, during, and after periods of demand. It requires recognizing that energy is not a single event but a continuous output that must be maintained through changing conditions.

When these two frames are placed side by side, the difference becomes clear. A system may be capable of producing a high peak of output while lacking the ability to sustain function afterward. Another system may never reach the same level of intensity, yet it may maintain steady, usable function across a longer span of time with fewer disruptions. In the first case, energy is high but unstable. In the second, energy is moderate but continuous.

This distinction is often overlooked because peaks are more noticeable than continuity. A surge of alertness draws attention. A stable baseline does not. The absence of disruption is less visible than the presence of intensity. As a result, continuity is often under-recognized as a defining feature of stability.

Peaks can be misleading because they isolate a moment from the process that surrounds it. A brief period of alertness may be followed by a decline that reduces function below baseline. A stretch of productive output may come at the cost of later fatigue, cognitive slowing, or changes in appetite. A period of heightened drive may be linked to transient stress activation rather than stable resource availability. In each case, the peak does not represent the system's overall condition. It represents a temporary configuration that may not be sustainable.

This does not mean that peaks are inherently problematic. They are a natural part of system behavior. Energy is not expected to remain flat across time. Variation is normal. What matters is how those variations are integrated into the broader pattern of output. A peak that emerges within a stable system will tend to resolve without significant disruption. A peak that emerges within an unstable system may be followed by a pronounced decline, requiring extended recovery or leading to compensatory responses.

The key limitation of peak-based interpretation is that it ignores what happens after the peak. It treats intensity as evidence of system stability without asking whether the output can be sustained, whether recovery will be proportionate, or whether the system is borrowing from future capacity to produce present output.

Continuity provides a more complete measure because it incorporates time. It reflects not just what the system can produce, but how it behaves across sequences of demand and recovery. It allows for variation while maintaining a focus on function. Stable energy does not require that output remains constant at every moment. It requires that output remains usable. This distinction is essential. Usability does not depend on intensity. It depends on whether the system can support ongoing activity without repeated breakdown.

Within this frame, stability is not defined by how elevated energy feels. It is defined by how consistently function can be maintained. A stable system may feel unremarkable in any single moment. It may not produce dramatic surges of alertness or unusually high output. Instead, it supports a steady progression of activity, with transitions that are smooth rather than abrupt and recoveries that are proportionate rather than prolonged.

This introduces an important clarification. Stability is not the same as flatness. A stable energy system is not one in which output remains identical across time. It is one in which variation occurs within a range that does not disrupt function. Energy may rise and fall in response to changing demands, inputs, and internal conditions. These changes are expected. What defines stability is that these fluctuations do not lead to repeated collapse, excessive volatility, or a loss of continuity.

Constant elevation is also not the goal. A system that remains in a persistently elevated state may be operating under sustained activation that is not indefinitely maintainable. Elevation without recovery can create its own form of instability. The aim is not to maximize intensity but to maintain alignment between output, capacity, and recovery.

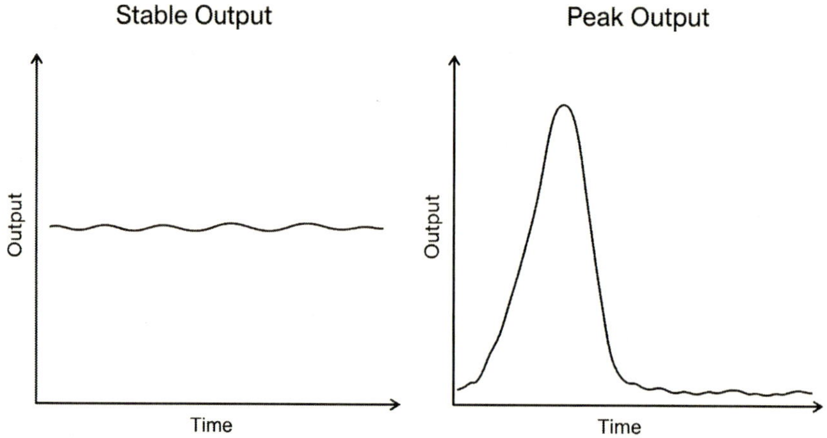

[Figure 2 — Stable Output vs Peak Output]

The contrast illustrated here emphasizes the difference between these two patterns. On one side, output rises sharply to a high level before declining, creating a visible peak followed by a drop. On the other, output remains within a moderate range but continues across time with minimal disruption. The visual contrast highlights the distinction. The higher line appears more impressive in isolation, but it does not persist. The moderate line, while less striking at any single point, maintains function across a longer duration. The figure makes visible what is otherwise difficult to observe when attention is drawn to peaks alone.

The Output Continuity Mechanism formalizes this distinction. It defines energy stability as the ability to sustain usable function across time rather than produce isolated peaks of output. Within this mechanism, the central question becomes whether the system can maintain function through sequences of demand without repeated interruption, collapse, or excessive recovery cost.

Several features emerge from this definition. Usable function becomes the primary reference point. Energy is not evaluated based on how it feels at its highest point, but on whether it supports ongoing activity. Continuity across demand becomes the structural requirement. The system must be able to respond to successive demands without degradation that accumulates into instability. Volatility is reduced, not by eliminating variation, but by preventing large swings that disrupt function. Collapses become less frequent and less severe. Recovery between demands becomes smoother, allowing the system to return to baseline without prolonged impairment. Dependence on compensation decreases, as the system relies less on mechanisms that temporarily elevate output at the expense of later stability.

This mechanism does not isolate energy from the rest of the system. It integrates energy into a network of interacting processes. Fuel availability influences whether output can be sustained. Signal coordination determines how resources are distributed and utilized. Recovery capacity defines how quickly the system can restore function after demand. Constraint load reflects the accumulation of factors that limit performance over time. Each of these elements contributes to whether continuity can be maintained.

The emphasis on continuity shifts the interpretive frame for common experiences. An energy crash is no longer viewed as an isolated event but as a disruption in continuity. Fatigue is not simply a reduction in intensity but a limitation in sustained function. Baseline drift reflects a gradual change in the system's ability to maintain output over time. Compensation appears as an attempt to restore function through temporary adjustments that may not support long-term stability.

This perspective also alters how variability is understood. Fluctuations in energy are not inherently problematic. They become meaningful when they interfere with continuity. A rise in energy that resolves without disruption fits within a stable pattern. A rise that leads to a pronounced decline introduces instability. The difference lies not in the presence of variation, but in its integration into the broader pattern of output.

The Output Continuity Mechanism therefore establishes a different standard for evaluating energy. It replaces the focus on peaks with a focus on patterns. It moves from isolated moments to sequences across time. It recognizes that energy is not a resource that can be judged by its highest expression, but a system output that must be interpreted through its behavior under changing conditions.

This mechanism becomes the lens through which the rest of the book is organized. Each subsequent concept can be understood in terms of its impact on continuity. Crashes become interruptions in sustained output. Fatigue reflects a reduction in the system's ability to maintain function. Baseline drift indicates a change in the level at which continuity can be preserved. Compensation reveals attempts to temporarily restore output when underlying continuity is compromised. Appetite, glucose, insulin, stress load, sleep, and recovery can then be understood by how they affect the system's ability to sustain function across time.

By establishing continuity as the governing frame, the chapter defines what it means to interpret energy as a system output. Energy is no longer treated as a target to be increased or a state to be maintained at a high level. It is understood as a reflection of how well the system can support ongoing function. The focus shifts from trying to elevate energy to understanding how it behaves.

This shift prepares the transition to the next mechanism. If energy is an output that must be interpreted through its continuity, then the question becomes how that output is experienced and recognized. The system produces energy as a functional capacity, but it is perceived as a felt state. The relationship between what the system generates and what is experienced introduces a new layer of complexity. The next chapter examines this relationship, where internal state becomes felt energy and interpretation begins to shape how output is understood.

Perception Mechanism

How internal state becomes felt energy.

Energy is felt before it is analyzed. A person does not first encounter energy as physiology, metabolic regulation, glucose movement, sleep architecture, stress response, hydration status, or recovery capacity. Those processes may be operating continuously, but they are not how energy first appears in ordinary experience. Energy arrives as sensation. It is felt as alertness, heaviness, fog, resistance, drive, fatigue, readiness, urgency, or lack of momentum.

This immediacy makes energy difficult to interpret. The feeling comes before explanation, and because it comes first, it often appears to explain itself. A clear morning may seem to mean that the system is ready. A heavy afternoon may seem to mean that something has failed. A period of fog may seem like lack of focus. A sudden urgency may seem like genuine capacity. A lack of momentum may seem like reluctance. The experience is so direct that it can be mistaken for a complete account of the system producing it.

This is the opening misreading of felt energy. Because the sensation is available, the sensation is often treated as the explanation.

The Perception Mechanism begins by separating experience from origin. Felt energy is real, but it is not self-explanatory. Fatigue is not imaginary because it is subjective. Heaviness is not unreal because it cannot be reduced to one visible measurement. Fog is not fake because it is difficult to quantify. Urgency is not meaningless because it is felt internally. These sensations are not illusions floating above the body. They are experiences generated through the body's interpretation of its own condition.

The issue is not whether the sensation is valid. The issue is whether the sensation, by itself, identifies the system state that produced it. A person may feel tired, but the feeling itself does not specify whether the dominant contributor is poor sleep, limited fuel access, glucose volatility, stress load, recovery debt, fluid balance, appetite signaling, current demand, prior exertion, or a combination of factors. The sensation is real as experience, but incomplete as explanation.

This distinction prevents two opposite errors. The first is dismissing felt energy as "just subjective," as though the fact that energy is experienced internally makes it less real. The second is treating felt energy as complete evidence of its cause, as though the body's final perception contains a full diagnostic map of the underlying system. Both errors flatten the mechanism. Felt energy is neither meaningless nor complete. It is a signal surface created from deeper regulatory activity.

The body is continuously interpreting internal state, but this interpretation is not conscious analysis. The body is not moving through a checklist, measuring each variable separately, and then producing a verbal conclusion. It is integrating signals. Fuel availability affects whether output can be supported. Glucose changes may alter alertness, hunger, urgency, steadiness, or fog. Sleep state changes the system receiving the day's demands, influencing readiness before the first demand is even encountered. Stress load may create activation while also increasing strain, producing a state that feels energetic in one layer and costly in another.

Hydration and fluid balance influence circulation, signaling, and physical ease. Appetite signals can change the sense of urgency, depletion, distraction, or internal pressure. Recovery capacity affects whether ordinary demand feels manageable or costly. Prior exertion changes the meaning of current effort because the system is not beginning from a neutral position. Current demand alters perception by increasing the amount of output required in the moment. Recent intake and fasting state influence fuel access, digestive load, and signal timing. Environmental demand can make the same internal state feel different by changing how much response is required. Circadian timing shapes alertness and readiness across the day, not as a rigid schedule, but as a background rhythm that influences how other signals are interpreted.

Perceived energy is therefore produced systemically. It is not the output of one isolated variable. The body does not provide separate sensations for every contributing layer. It does not give one clean feeling for glucose movement, another for sleep debt, another for stress load, another for hydration, another for appetite pressure, another for recovery capacity, and another for fuel access. Instead, those layers are compressed into one felt state.

That compression is why felt energy can seem simpler than it is. A person feels fatigue, fog, heaviness, urgency, alertness, resistance, drive, readiness, or lack of momentum as a single condition. The simplicity of the feeling can hide the complexity of the system producing it. What arrives as one experience may reflect many internal inputs converging at once.

Fatigue may come from poor sleep, accumulated stress, glucose volatility, recovery limitation, fluid instability, prior exertion, or load exceeding capacity. Alertness may come from recovery, stress activation, environmental demand, fuel access, or short-term compensation. Heaviness may reflect reduced readiness, digestive load, poor recovery, or a conservation response. Urgency may feel like readiness, but it may also reflect activation under strain. Fog may reflect sleep debt, glucose patterning, stress load, or accumulated cognitive demand. These are not diagnoses. They are examples of why one felt state cannot be assumed to have one origin.

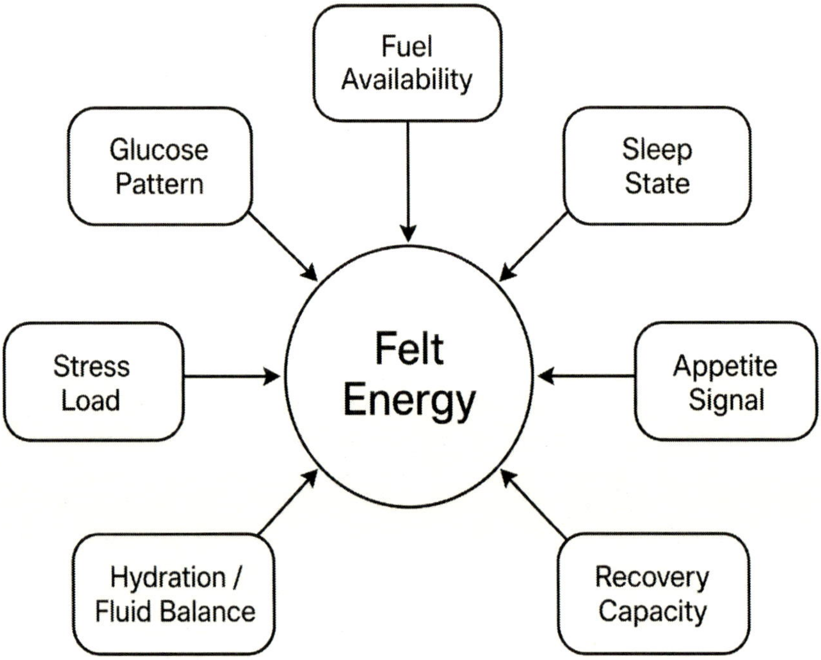

[Figure 3 — Internal State to Felt Energy]

Prior state changes the meaning of the present moment. The same visible condition may feel different depending on what came before it. A normal task may feel manageable after recovery and heavy after poor sleep. The task itself may not have changed, but the system receiving the task has. The same meal may feel stabilizing in one context and sluggish in another. The same fasting period may feel clear in one condition and draining in another. The same stressor may feel activating at one point and overwhelming at another. The same level of activity may feel light when capacity is high and costly when capacity is low.

This is context dependence. The body does not interpret current demand from an empty baseline. It interprets the present through accumulated context. A condition does not arrive into an empty system. A meal does not arrive into an empty system. A task does not arrive into an empty system. A fasting window does not arrive into an empty system. A stressor does not arrive into an empty system. Each arrives into a system already shaped by prior sleep, prior intake, prior exertion, prior stress, prior recovery, prior appetite signaling, and prior demand.

This matters because energy perception is not simply a reaction to the present input. It is a response to the present input as filtered through existing state. Prior state affects tolerance, interpretation, and perceived cost. A demand that would be absorbed easily under one condition may feel disproportionate under another. A signal that would be barely noticeable when the system is stable may become dominant when constraint load is higher. The same event can therefore generate different felt energy because the system context has changed.

This explains why energy can feel inconsistent even when visible behavior appears consistent. A person may follow a similar schedule, eat at similar times, perform similar work, face similar demands, or sleep for a similar duration, yet experience different energy states across days. From the outside, the pattern appears stable. Internally, the system may not be operating from the same conditions.

Sleep duration may look similar while sleep quality differs. Stress load may differ even when the calendar looks unchanged. Glucose movement may differ even when meals appear similar. Recovery debt may accumulate even when activity appears ordinary. Appetite pressure may shift even when intake timing looks consistent. Fluid balance may differ even when routine looks familiar. Prior demand may leave a residual load that is not visible in the present day's schedule. The question "I did the same thing, so why do I feel different?" often reflects this gap between visible behavior and internal state.

Visible consistency does not guarantee internal consistency. The body is not only responding to what can be seen from the outside. It is responding to the condition of the system beneath the visible pattern. Energy perception brings that internal condition into experience, but it does so through compression. It gives a felt state, not a full explanation.

The Perception Mechanism explains how internal system conditions are translated into felt energy states. It includes signal integration, composite perception, prior-state influence, context dependence, real but incomplete sensation, and interpretation of system status. Energy is not merely produced and then noticed. It is produced, interpreted, and felt. The feeling is part of the system's communication, but it is not the entire system.

This mechanism protects energy from simplistic mindset explanations. Fatigue is not laziness. Heaviness is not weakness. Fog is not simply lack of focus. Resistance is not automatically a character problem. Urgency is not always true readiness. Motivation may be part of the experience, but it is not the full mechanism. A felt state may influence behavior, but it should not be reduced to character, discipline, attitude, or willpower.

At the same time, the mechanism does not require a rigid separation between mind and body. Cognition, emotion, behavior, expectation, and physiology interact. The point is not to remove experience from physiology or to claim that every felt state has only one physical explanation. The point is to prevent one-layer interpretations. Perception is one way physiology becomes experience. Felt energy is where internal regulation becomes available to awareness.

This connects directly back to the Energy Continuity Mechanism. Chapter 1 established that stable energy is continuity rather than intensity. Energy stability is not defined by isolated peaks of output, but by the system's ability to sustain usable function across time. Chapter 2 adds that continuity must be interpreted through felt experience. A system may produce output, but the person experiences that output as readiness, fog, fatigue, resistance, steadiness, urgency, or momentum.

Energy continuity describes the stability of functional output across time. Perception describes how that output is experienced from within the system. Together, they prevent two interpretive errors. The first is judging energy only by visible output, as though function can be understood without felt state. The second is treating felt energy as a complete explanation, as though the sensation itself identifies the underlying cause.

Inconsistent energy is not necessarily irrational. It may reflect changing internal state. The body may be responding to prior sleep, accumulated demand, glucose dynamics, recovery debt, stress load, appetite signals, hydration and fluid balance, fuel availability, circadian timing, or the interaction among these conditions. What feels like unpredictability may be a perception of system variation that has not yet been interpreted structurally.

The Perception Mechanism therefore deepens the foundation of the book. Energy is not a target to force upward, a motivational state to manufacture, or a simple reflection of attitude. It is a regulated output that becomes experience through perception. That perception is real, but it must be interpreted through the system that produced it.

If felt energy is a perception of internal state, the next question is why that perception changes across the day. Energy rises, falls, shifts, and changes because the system is continuously responding to demand, recovery, fuel access, signal coordination, and constraint load. The next chapter examines that movement through the Variability Mechanism, distinguishing normal daily variation from instability.

Variability Mechanism

Why energy rises, falls, and changes across the day.

Stable energy is often imagined as a straight line. In that picture, the ideal day would feel evenly powered from beginning to end, with the same level of alertness, readiness, and functional capacity available at every hour. Any dip would appear suspicious. Any shift would appear like a failure of regulation. Any fatigue would be interpreted as instability.

That image does not describe how energy behaves in a living system.

Energy is not supposed to remain identical across the day. The body is continuously responding to changing conditions. Demand rises and falls. Fuel availability changes. Sleep state transitions into wakefulness. Stress load increases or resolves. Appetite signals shift. Meals alter digestive and regulatory activity. Circadian timing changes the background state of alertness. Recovery capacity is used and restored. Prior exertion changes the cost of present output. Because the system is dynamic, the experience of energy is dynamic as well.

This means that movement itself is not instability. Energy may rise in the morning as the system transitions into wakefulness and begins responding to daily demand. It may shift after meals as digestion, fuel availability, insulin signaling, glucose movement, and appetite regulation change the internal environment. It may soften in the afternoon as accumulated demand meets changing timing and recovery bandwidth. It may decline toward evening as the system moves closer to restoration. It may include lower-output windows that allow continuity to be preserved rather than broken.

The important distinction is not whether energy changes. The important distinction is what kind of change is occurring and what that change does to continuity.

Stability does not mean flatness. A stable system can move. Energy can rise during demand, soften during recovery, dip after meals, shift with timing, or decline toward the end of the day without automatically indicating dysfunction. Stability means that these movements remain within a range that preserves usable function. The system can change state without losing coherence. It can respond to demand without collapsing. It can recover from dips without excessive cost. It can transition between higher and lower output without repeated disruption.

Stable energy can include mild dips. It can include natural fatigue. It can include transitions between more alert and less alert states. It can include recovery windows. It can include different energy states across the day. The presence of variation does not contradict stability because stability is not identical sameness. Stability is regulated movement within tolerable limits.

This range-based view matters because it prevents the reader from mistaking every fluctuation for a problem. A dip is not automatically a crash. A softer period is not automatically instability. A lower-output window is not automatically failure. Energy becomes meaningful when it is interpreted by pattern, recovery, and continuity. The question is whether function remains usable and whether recovery remains proportionate.

Morning activation is one example of normal rhythm. As the system shifts from sleep into wakefulness, output often changes. The body is no longer maintaining the same state required for sleep. It is preparing for upright movement, attention, interaction, and external demand. Energy may rise as the system organizes around waking function. This rise does not need to be dramatic to be meaningful. It reflects transition into a different mode of operation.

Post-meal shifts show another form of normal movement. Eating changes internal conditions. Digestion begins. Nutrients enter circulation. Insulin signaling adjusts distribution and storage. Glucose movement changes. Appetite signals begin to resolve or reorganize. Some people may feel steadier after eating in one context and heavier in another, but the broader point is that the system state has changed. A shift in energy after eating is not inherently unstable. It becomes more meaningful when the shift is sharp, disruptive, recurrent, or difficult to recover from.

Afternoon dips can also fit within ordinary rhythm. By later portions of the day, demand has accumulated. Attention, movement, emotional processing, work, environmental load, and prior decisions may have drawn on available capacity. Circadian timing may also shift the background level of alertness. Fuel patterns and recovery bandwidth may be different from the morning state. A softening of energy in this context does not automatically indicate a broken system. It may reflect normal movement across the day.

Evening fatigue is similar. Some decline toward evening may represent a transition toward recovery rather than a sign of instability. A system that never moves toward lower output may not be stable; it may be persistently activated. Recovery requires periods in which output can decrease. Lower energy at the end of the day may be part of the rhythm by which continuity is preserved across longer time horizons.

Recovery windows are therefore not interruptions by default. A lower-output period can serve the stability of the whole pattern if it allows the system to restore function. The issue is not that output temporarily decreases. The issue is whether the decrease is integrated, recoverable, and proportionate, or whether it becomes prolonged, disruptive, and difficult to reverse.

Variation becomes instability when it begins to interfere with continuity. The system is not unstable because it moves. It becomes unstable when movement becomes too sharp, too recurrent, too costly, or too poorly recovered. Sharp drops, jagged swings, repeated crashes, prolonged recovery after dips, inability to return to baseline, progressive baseline decline, repeated need for compensation, high volatility after ordinary demands, or energy changes that disrupt appetite, focus, movement, or daily function all indicate a different pattern.

Instability is not defined by one dip. It is defined by pattern, recurrence, disruption, and recovery cost. A single lower-energy period after unusual demand may be understandable within the larger rhythm. A repeated collapse after ordinary demand suggests a more important continuity issue. A temporary decline that resolves cleanly belongs to one pattern. A decline that lingers, lowers the next baseline, or requires repeated compensation belongs to another.

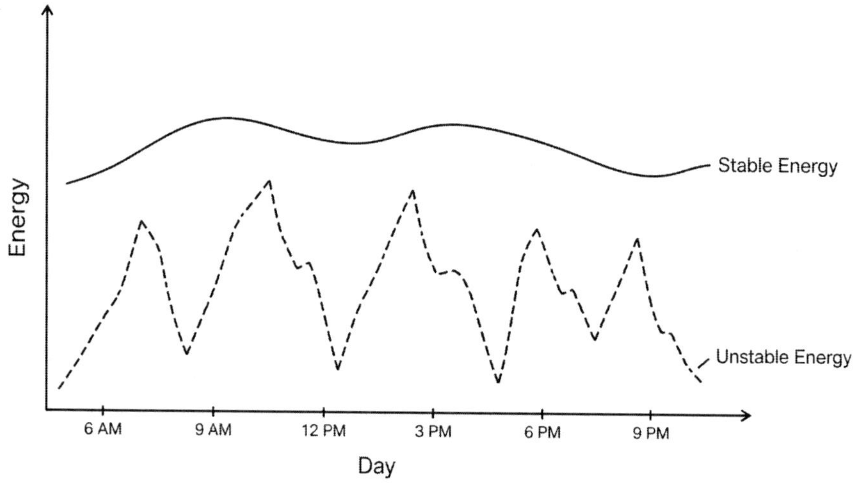

[Figure 4 — Normal Rhythm vs Instability]

Smooth variation can preserve continuity. Energy may rise and fall without breaking the system's functional pattern. A stable rhythm is characterized by transitions that are not abrupt, dips that remain recoverable, demand responses that do not produce collapse, recovery periods that restore function, variation that remains within tolerable range, and output that continues without repeated disruption.

This is why constant elevation is not the standard. A person does not need to feel equally energetic all day for the pattern to be stable. Equal output at every hour would not reflect the actual demands of a changing system. The body does not remain in one regulatory state. It shifts in response to timing, intake, activity, stress, rest, and recovery. A stable rhythm allows those shifts without allowing them to fragment the day into repeated interruptions.

Smooth variation has a different quality from volatility. It may be noticeable, but it is not destabilizing. It may include lower points, but those lower points do not erase function. It may include transitions, but those transitions do not require excessive recovery. It may include fatigue, but fatigue appears in proportion to demand and timing rather than as an abrupt collapse that disrupts continuity.

Jagged variation signals lower continuity. Jaggedness includes sudden rises and drops, pronounced crashes, unpredictable volatility, sharp post-demand declines, or repeated energy interruption. A system may still produce moments of high output within a jagged pattern, but those peaks do not prove stability. This connects directly back to the Output Continuity Mechanism. High output in isolation says little about the pattern surrounding it. A peak followed by steep decline may represent intensity without continuity.

The problem with jagged variation is not merely that energy changes quickly. The problem is that rapid shifts can fragment function. A person may feel capable for a short window and then lose usable output. A demand that appears manageable at first may be followed by a disproportionate drop. A period of activation may require an extended recovery. A moment of alertness may be followed by fog, heaviness, appetite disruption, or resistance. These patterns matter because they affect the ability to sustain function across time.

Recurrent variation matters more than isolated variation. One low-energy period does not define the system. A dip after one unusual demand may reflect the cost of that demand. A recurring dip after ordinary demand suggests lower tolerance. A single crash may reflect a specific context. Repeated crashes suggest a continuity problem. A temporary decline may be recoverable. Progressive drift suggests a changing baseline.

Pattern recognition changes interpretation. Without recurrence, every energy movement can appear equally important. With recurrence, the system's behavior becomes clearer. The question shifts from "Did energy dip?" to "How often does this dip occur, under what conditions, how disruptive is it, and how well does recovery follow?" This creates a more stable interpretive frame. It does not exaggerate ordinary rhythm, and it does not dismiss repeated disruption.

Recovery separates normal rhythm from instability. A stable system can move away from baseline and return without excessive cost. It can rise to meet demand and then soften without collapsing. It can experience a dip and then restore usable function. It can shift between states without requiring repeated compensation to maintain basic output.

Variation becomes more important when recovery is delayed, incomplete, or dependent on compensation. Normal rhythm means output shifts and then recovers. Disruptive variation means output drops and recovery is delayed. A crash pattern means output falls sharply. A drift pattern means baseline gradually lowers. A compensation pattern means output is temporarily restored while future stability is strained. These patterns are not fully developed here, but they become easier to understand once ordinary variation has been separated from instability.

This distinction prepares the next stage of the book. Crashes, drift, and compensation are not simply stronger versions of normal variation. They are specific patterns of continuity disruption. A crash interrupts output sharply. Drift lowers the functional baseline over time. Compensation temporarily preserves output by increasing strain elsewhere in the system.

Each pattern depends on the same central question: what happens to continuity when energy moves?

The Variability Mechanism explains how energy moves within a range across the day and why variation itself is not the same as instability. It includes natural rhythm, range-based stability, tolerable variation, disruptive variability, recovery cost, and continuity impact. Energy movement must be interpreted by pattern, not by the mere presence of change.

This mechanism completes the opening foundation of the book. Chapter 1 established that stable energy is continuity rather than intensity. Chapter 2 explained that felt energy is real but not self-explanatory. Chapter 3 now clarifies that energy naturally rises, falls, and changes across the day. These movements are not automatically signs of instability. They become meaningful through rhythm, range, recurrence, disruption, and recovery cost.

Once normal variation is separated from instability, the book can examine the mechanisms that make energy drop sharply, decline gradually, or require compensation to maintain output. The next section turns toward the conditions that support energy before those patterns appear: fuel availability, fuel-state transitions, and the conversion processes that allow functional output to continue across changing demand.

Fuel Availability Mechanism

Energy depends on accessible fuel, not just intake.

Energy problems are often interpreted as fuel quantity problems. If energy feels low, the assumption is often that more fuel is needed. If food has already been eaten, the assumption is often that energy should now be available. If stored fuel exists in the body, the assumption is often that the system should be able to draw from it whenever output is required. If fuel is circulating, the assumption is often that functional energy should be stable.

This treats energy as an inventory problem. Under that frame, the main question becomes whether fuel exists somewhere in the system. Food has entered. Storage is present. Fuel is moving. Therefore, output should follow. But daily energy does not operate through inventory alone. Fuel must move through regulation before it becomes stable function. It must be accessible, timed, coordinated, and matched to demand. Its existence matters, but existence is only one layer.

Energy depends on accessible fuel, not just fuel presence. Fuel can exist without being accessible. Fuel can be accessible without being well-timed. Fuel can circulate without being smoothly used. Fuel can be present while still being poorly matched to the demand placed on the system. This distinction does not turn fuel into a moral category or a behavioral verdict. It simply separates fuel quantity from fuel availability.

Intake is the beginning, not the output. Food entering the body is not the same as functional energy. Intake begins a regulatory process.

Food must be digested, absorbed, regulated, distributed, stored, released, circulated, taken up, converted, and matched to demand before it can support stable output. These steps do not occur outside context. They occur inside a system already shaped by prior state.

That prior state matters because food does not enter an empty system. It enters a body already influenced by prior intake, fasting state, stress load, sleep state, glucose pattern, insulin signaling, appetite state, digestive demand, recovery capacity, and current demand. The same intake can therefore be handled differently under different conditions. The material entering the system may be similar, but the system receiving it may not be similar.

A meal can add material without immediately creating stable functional energy. It may support steadier output in one context and contribute to heaviness, fog, urgency, or volatility in another. The difference is not explained by intake alone. It depends on timing, regulatory response, demand, and the system's capacity to distribute and use what has entered. Eating answers the question of whether fuel entered the system. It does not answer whether fuel became usable in the right form, at the right time, and in proportion to demand.

Stored fuel adds a second layer. Storage represents potential energy in the system. It means the body has reserves, but reserves are not the same as active access. Stored fuel must be signaled for release, mobilized, transported, routed, taken up, converted, and matched to demand. Storage is capacity. Availability is deployment.

This distinction is often misread because stored energy appears to imply immediate access. If energy exists somewhere in reserve, it may seem as though the system should be able to use it directly whenever needed. But the body does not operate as an open container where reserves automatically flow into function. Stored fuel is regulated. It is held, released, conserved, or mobilized depending on signals, state, and demand.

The presence of stored fuel does not mean that energy will feel stable, immediate, or easily accessible in every condition. Energy instability can occur when stored fuel exists but access is delayed, constrained, mistimed, poorly coordinated, mismatched to demand, or dependent on compensation. This is not a weight-loss argument and not a fat-storage argument. It is an access argument. The question is not whether energy exists somewhere in the system. The question is whether the system can make that energy usable when function requires it.

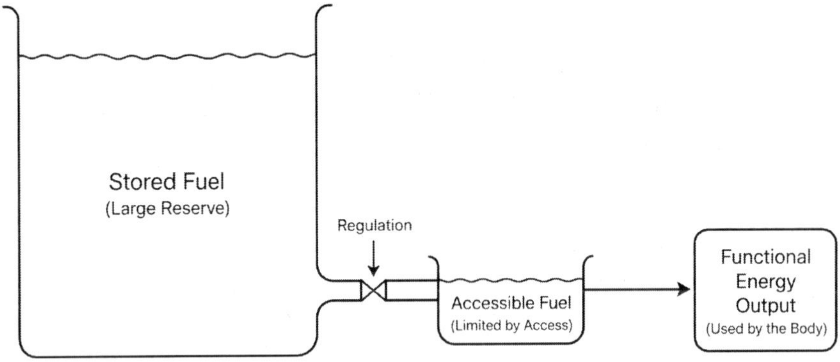

[Figure 5 — Stored Fuel vs Accessible Fuel]

Circulating fuel is another layer, but it is still not the same as continuity. Fuel may be present in the bloodstream, yet the system still has to coordinate uptake, distribution, regulation, timing, demand matching, and conversion support. Circulation answers whether fuel is moving through the system. It does not fully answer whether output can be sustained.

This matters because circulating fuel can be poorly timed or poorly matched. Fuel may appear rapidly but fail to remain steady. It may be available during low demand but less available when demand rises. It may rise in a way that creates volatility rather than continuity. It may depend on compensation instead of smooth regulation. It may be present while recovery state or stress load limits usable output.

In those cases, the issue is not simple absence. Fuel is present, but the pattern does not support stable function. Circulating fuel may help meet a moment of demand, yet fail to preserve continuity across time. It may produce a temporary rise without a durable pattern. It may move through the system without being coordinated smoothly enough to support ordinary function without interruption.

Fuel availability is therefore an active process. Fuel must be present, but it must also be accessible. Stored fuel must be mobilized when needed. Incoming fuel must be regulated. Circulating fuel must be transported and taken up. Fuel must be converted into usable output. Timing must match demand. Availability is not a passive state. It is a coordinated sequence.

This is the boundary between Chapter 4 and Chapter 5. Chapter 4 is about access. Chapter 5 is about conversion. Fuel availability means the system can make fuel reachable for function. Energy conversion means the system can turn reachable fuel into usable work. Availability is necessary, but it is not the final step.

Fuel access changes because the regulatory state of the system changes. Insulin state helps coordinate distribution, storage, and access. Insulin is not a villain or an obstacle in this frame. It is a coordination signal that helps determine how fuel is routed after intake and how availability changes across fed and fasted conditions. It influences whether fuel is directed toward immediate use, storage, or later release within a broader regulatory pattern.

Fasting state changes the source and timing of available fuel. When incoming fuel is absent, the system relies more heavily on stored fuel and mobilized reserves. This does not make fasting inherently beneficial or harmful. It changes the regulatory context. The meaning of that shift depends on prior state, demand, stress load, recovery capacity, and the system's ability to move between fuel sources without excessive strain.

Prior intake affects current availability because fuel handling has a history. Recent meals can influence circulating patterns, digestive load, appetite state, insulin signaling, glucose movement, and timing. The present energy state is not produced only by the present moment. It reflects the regulatory consequences of what came before.

Activity demand changes how much fuel must be accessible and when. Higher demand requires more coordination between supply, transport, uptake, and conversion. If demand rises faster than accessible fuel can support it, energy may feel strained even when fuel exists elsewhere. Lower demand may require less immediate access, but still depends on smooth regulation to preserve continuity.

Stress load can also alter fuel access. Stress may change activation, urgency, demand, and regulatory priorities. It may temporarily increase perceived energy while also increasing system cost. Under higher stress load, fuel handling may be shaped less by smooth continuity and more by immediate response. The result can be a state that feels temporarily activated but less stable across time.

Metabolic flexibility affects whether the system can shift between fuel sources as conditions change. When switching is smoother, continuity has more support. When switching is constrained, energy may become more vulnerable to timing, demand, and prior state. A system with fewer accessible options may rely more heavily on one source or one pattern, making transitions more costly.

Recovery state determines whether available fuel can support function without excessive strain. Fuel access alone does not eliminate recovery limits. A system carrying recovery debt may have fuel present and even accessible, yet still experience heaviness, resistance, or reduced output because the limiting factor is not only supply. It is the capacity to translate supply into function without adding further strain.

These access conditions show why fuel availability is not fixed. It changes with the regulatory state of the system. The same amount of intake, the same stored reserve, or the same circulating fuel pattern may support different energy outcomes depending on insulin state, fasting state, prior intake, activity demand, stress load, metabolic flexibility, and recovery state. Fuel access is not a static property. It is a moving relationship between supply, regulation, and demand.

This creates the core interpretive gap: fuel can be present in the system without being available to the person as stable daily energy. "I ate, so I should have energy" overlooks digestion, distribution, timing, demand matching, and system state. "I have stored energy, so I should be able to access it" overlooks mobilization, regulation, signaling, and timing. "Fuel is circulating, so output should be stable" overlooks uptake, coordination, recovery state, stress load, and conversion constraints. "Low energy means fuel is absent" overlooks access limitations, volatility, mismatch, stress load, recovery debt, and signal coordination.

These are common interpretive shortcuts, not failures of reasoning. They arise because fuel is easy to imagine as material and harder to see as regulation. Fuel presence describes what exists. Fuel availability describes what can be used. The difference matters because energy stability depends on use, not existence alone.

This connects directly to the Energy Continuity Mechanism. Stable energy requires usable output across time. If fuel access is smooth, energy may remain within a tolerable range even as demand changes. If fuel access is delayed, volatile, constrained, or mismatched, energy may become unstable. The system may still contain fuel, but continuity may be interrupted because access does not match functional need.

Fuel availability can sit beneath many later energy experiences. A dip may reflect a temporary mismatch between available fuel and demand. A crash may reflect a sharper interruption in functional supply. Urgency may emerge when the system signals need before usable output is restored. Heaviness may appear when fuel handling, digestive load, or recovery constraints reduce readiness. Fog may emerge when fuel dynamics and signal coordination fail to support stable function. Compensation may temporarily restore output when smooth access is not available. Drift may develop when repeated mismatches gradually lower the functional baseline.

The Fuel Availability Mechanism explains the gap between fuel that exists in the body and fuel that is usable for stable functional output. It includes intake, storage, circulation, mobilization, transport, access, regulation, demand matching, and continuity impact. Energy depends on whether fuel can become usable at the right time, in the right form, and in proportion to demand.

This mechanism opens the physical foundation of the book. The first three chapters established how energy should be interpreted: as continuity rather than intensity, as felt but not self-explanatory, and as variable without automatically being unstable. Chapter 4 adds the first fuel layer beneath that interpretation. Daily energy depends not only on whether fuel exists, but on whether the system can make fuel reachable for function.

Fuel availability is necessary, but it is not the final step. Accessible fuel must still become usable work. Chapter 5 turns to the Energy Conversion Mechanism, where the book examines how accessible fuel becomes functional output through conversion, cellular demand, oxygen delivery, recovery state, and system constraints.

Energy Conversion Mechanism

How accessible fuel becomes usable functional output.

Chapter 4 established that energy depends on accessible fuel, not just fuel presence. Food intake, stored fuel, and circulating substrates do not automatically create stable daily energy. Fuel must become available, mobilized, transported, coordinated, and matched to demand. Chapter 5 adds the next distinction: accessible fuel is still not the same as usable functional output.

The common assumption is that once fuel is available, energy should follow. If the system can reach fuel, if fuel can circulate, if stored reserves can be mobilized, then function should become steady. This assumption is understandable because access feels like the missing step. Once fuel is no longer merely present but reachable, it seems as though the system should be able to convert that reachability into energy without further complication.

But fuel availability describes access. Energy conversion describes use. Available fuel is not the same as usable energy.

Fuel can be reachable without becoming stable function. Accessible fuel means the system can bring fuel into a position where it may support output. Usable energy requires more. Fuel must be taken up, processed, coordinated, and converted into work under the conditions currently present in the system. Access moves fuel toward function, but conversion determines whether that fuel can become functional output.

This distinction explains why fuel can appear sufficient while energy still feels limited. A person may have eaten and still feel heavy. Fuel may be circulating and still not feel like usable energy. Stored fuel may be mobilized while output still feels strained. The system may have supply, but the conditions required to translate supply into function may be constrained. These examples do not identify one cause. They show why access is not the final layer.

Chapter 4 asked whether fuel can become reachable. Chapter 5 asks whether reachable fuel can become functional output. The difference matters because daily energy is not produced by fuel alone. It is produced by fuel moving through a conversion system that must coordinate cellular use, oxygen delivery, circulation, current demand, recovery state, stress load, and system tolerance.

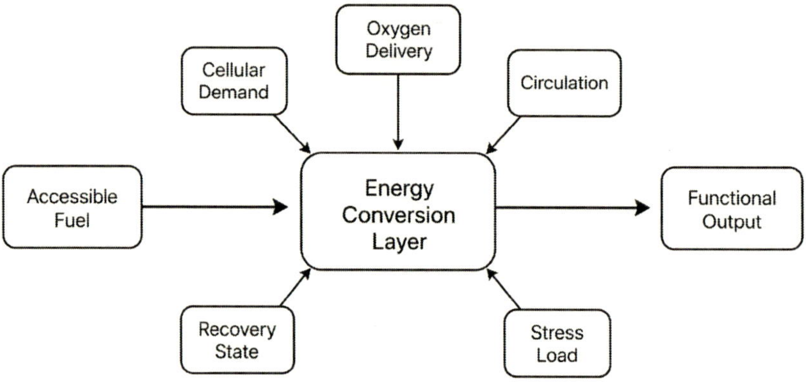

[Figure 6 — Energy Conversion Layer]

Conversion includes cellular processes, but daily energy is not explained by cells alone. A narrow view would treat energy as though fuel simply arrives at the cellular level and becomes output automatically. That view is incomplete because cells operate inside a larger physiological environment. The body must coordinate fuel access, cellular uptake, oxygen delivery, circulation, mitochondrial function, current demand, recovery state, stress load, illness or immune load, prior exertion, sleep state, fluid balance, and signaling support.

This means conversion is systemic. Cellular work matters, but it is not isolated from the conditions that support it. Fuel must be available to the tissue. Circulation must help deliver what is needed. Oxygen must be available to support conversion. Demand must be matched by capacity. Recovery state must allow output without excessive strain. Stress load must not distort the system's priorities so severely that available fuel cannot translate smoothly into usable function.

Mitochondria can be understood as part of the cellular conversion layer, where fuel availability is translated into usable energy for cellular work. They matter because conversion has to occur within cells. But mitochondria should not be separated from the system around them or treated as a magic switch for energy. They are not an isolated explanation for every form of fatigue, nor are they a shortcut concept that bypasses the rest of physiology.

Mitochondria operate inside a context shaped by oxygen delivery, fuel availability, cellular demand, stress load, sleep state, illness, inflammation, recovery state, circulation, and signaling conditions. If those surrounding layers are constrained, the conversion layer may also be constrained. The issue is not simply whether mitochondria exist or whether fuel exists. The issue is whether the whole environment supports the translation of accessible fuel into sustained functional output.

This broader frame protects the chapter from reducing energy to one cellular feature. The conversion layer matters, but it cannot be separated from the conditions supporting it. A cell may need fuel, but it also depends on delivery, clearance, signaling, and demand. A tissue may require output, but output depends on whether the system can support that demand without creating strain that interrupts continuity.

Fuel conversion also depends on oxygen delivery and circulation. Fuel alone is not enough. Oxygen delivery helps support the conversion of fuel into usable work. Circulation helps deliver what tissues need and remove what must be cleared. These processes are not separate from daily energy; they are part of the infrastructure that allows fuel to become function.

Demand determines how much output is required and when. A low-demand state requires less immediate conversion capacity. A higher-demand state requires more coordination among supply, oxygen delivery, circulation, cellular uptake, and conversion. If demand rises faster than the system can coordinate those layers, energy may feel strained even when fuel is available. The limiting factor is not necessarily absence of fuel. It may be the system's ability to convert available fuel at the rate and stability required by the moment.

This is where conversion becomes a continuity issue. A system may manage conversion adequately under low demand but struggle when demand increases. It may support output briefly but not sustain it. It may convert enough fuel for a short interval, then require prolonged recovery. It may maintain function only by increasing strain elsewhere. In each case, the question is not only whether fuel is present or accessible. The question is whether conversion can keep pace with functional need.

This also explains why available fuel may feel different depending on the type of demand placed on the system. Physical demand, cognitive demand, emotional demand, immune demand, and environmental demand do not all draw on the system in the same way. Each requires coordination across fuel access, oxygen delivery, circulation, signaling, and recovery capacity. A person may have enough available fuel for ordinary background function but experience strain when demand becomes more concentrated, sustained, or layered. The issue is not simply that the system has run out of fuel. The issue may be that conversion has to occur under a higher coordination burden.

This coordination burden matters because energy is experienced as usable function, not as fuel chemistry. Fuel may be present, but if the system has to work harder to deliver oxygen, circulate substrates, support cellular uptake, manage stress activation, and recover from prior output, the resulting experience may be fatigue rather than readiness. The body may still be producing energy at a cellular level, but the cost of maintaining functional output may be higher. In that condition, available fuel does not translate cleanly into available daily energy.

Conversion tolerance describes the system's ability to turn available fuel into usable output under current conditions without excessive strain, volatility, or delayed recovery. It is not a fixed trait. It changes with state. The same accessible fuel may feel sufficient in one context and insufficient in another because the system's conversion conditions have changed.

Conversion tolerance may be reduced by poor sleep, illness, excessive stress, under-recovery, high demand, prior exertion, inflammatory load, inadequate recovery windows, or accumulated strain. These are general constraints, not diagnoses. Their significance is structural: they change the system receiving the fuel. When tolerance is lower, the body may have access to fuel while still finding it costly to translate that fuel into stable output.

Sleep state is one example. A system emerging from poor sleep may have fuel available, but the ability to coordinate output may be reduced. Stress load is another. Stress may increase activation while also raising the cost of maintaining function. Illness or immune load may redirect resources toward defense and repair, changing how output is experienced. Prior exertion may leave the system with available fuel but lower tolerance for additional demand. Under-recovery may make conversion feel less smooth because the system is carrying unresolved cost.

This explains why available fuel may feel different across contexts. Fuel that supports function under one condition may not produce the same felt energy under another. The difference is not always the fuel itself. It may be conversion tolerance, demand level, recovery state, oxygen delivery, circulation, stress load, or accumulated strain. Available fuel is filtered through the system's current capacity to use it.

Conversion can therefore become constrained even when fuel is present and accessible. Fuel may be available, but output feels heavy. Fuel may be available, but fatigue remains. Fuel may be available, but recovery after demand is slow. Fuel may be available, but the system cannot sustain output smoothly. Fuel may be available, but stress or poor sleep limits tolerance. These patterns do not mean fuel availability is irrelevant. They mean fuel availability is only one layer.

If conversion is constrained, adding more available fuel may not produce proportionate output. This is not an eating instruction or a behavioral rule. It is a mechanism distinction. Supply matters, but supply does not override every other constraint. The system still has to convert what is available into work, and that conversion depends on the state of the whole system.

The Energy Conversion Mechanism connects directly back to the Energy Continuity Mechanism. Stable energy requires more than fuel access. It requires conversion stability across time. If conversion is smooth, accessible fuel can support usable output without excessive strain. If conversion is constrained, daily energy may become unstable even when fuel is available.

Conversion constraints can contribute to heaviness, fog, fatigue, dips, delayed recovery, reduced tolerance, compensation, or drift. Heaviness may appear when the system has supply but cannot translate it easily into output. Fog may reflect a mismatch between demand and the system's ability to support stable function. Fatigue may remain when conversion conditions are limited by recovery state or accumulated strain. Dips may occur when conversion cannot keep pace with demand. Delayed recovery may indicate that the cost of output exceeded current tolerance. Compensation may temporarily preserve function when conversion is less stable. Drift may develop when repeated conversion strain gradually lowers baseline output.

These later patterns are not fully explained here, but they depend partly on the distinction this chapter establishes. Energy instability cannot be understood only by asking whether fuel exists or whether it is accessible. It must also ask whether the system can convert accessible fuel into usable function with enough stability to preserve continuity.

The Energy Conversion Mechanism explains how accessible fuel becomes usable functional output. It includes fuel access, cellular uptake, oxygen delivery, circulation, mitochondrial function, current demand, recovery state, stress load, conversion tolerance, and continuity impact. Available fuel does not automatically feel like available energy because the system must still convert it into usable output.

Chapter 4 explained access. Chapter 5 explained conversion. Together, they form the first physical foundation beneath daily energy: fuel must become reachable, and reachable fuel must become work. But even when fuel is available and conversion is possible, energy may still change as the system shifts between fuel states. Chapter 6 turns to the Transition Mechanism, where the book examines why energy may rise, fall, or feel unstable during shifts between glucose-dominant and fat-dominant conditions.

Transition Mechanism

Energy shifts during fuel switching between glucose and fat.

Energy may feel stable in one part of the day and unstable in another even when nothing dramatic has happened. A person may feel steady after eating but strained between meals. They may feel clear during one fasting window and foggy during another. They may feel ordinary at rest but unstable when activity, stress, or delayed intake changes the fuel state. The visible day may not appear unusual, yet the internal experience shifts.

The point is not that one state is right and another is wrong. The point is that energy often becomes unstable during the movement between states.

Energy instability often appears in the transition between fuel states, not because one fuel state is inherently wrong. This distinction keeps the chapter centered on movement rather than hierarchy. The issue is not whether the body is using glucose or fat in some absolute way. The issue is whether the system can move between changing conditions without interrupting functional output.

The body does not stay in one fuel state. Fuel reliance changes with feeding, fasting, sleep, waking, rest, activity, stress, prior intake, current demand, and recovery state. Daily energy is therefore not supported by a static fuel condition. It is supported by the system's ability to move across fuel conditions while preserving continuity.

A stable system is not one that avoids fuel shifts. It is one that shifts without repeatedly losing usable output. Movement itself is normal. The instability appears when movement becomes costly, delayed, volatile, or poorly coordinated.

The fed state is not simply "food is present." It is a regulatory condition. Food entering the body initiates digestion and absorption, but it also changes glucose movement, insulin signaling, storage, distribution, appetite signaling, and demand matching. The system must decide how incoming material will be routed, what will be used immediately, what will be stored, and how current output will be supported while those processes unfold.

Because the fed state is regulatory, feeding is not automatically stabilizing or destabilizing. In one context, incoming fuel may support smoother output. In another, the same general state may involve heaviness, fog, volatility, or appetite-energy mismatch. The difference is not explained by food presence alone. It depends on prior state, stress load, sleep state, current demand, recovery capacity, and the system's ability to coordinate incoming fuel with ongoing function.

The fasting state is also not simply "food is absent." It is a regulatory condition involving stored fuel mobilization, internal fuel access, signal adjustment, appetite pressure, stress interaction, demand matching, and reliance on reserves. The absence of incoming fuel changes the system's source of supply, but it does not remove the need for coordination. Stored fuel must become accessible. Demand must still be met. Signals must adjust to the changed condition.

Fasting is therefore not automatically stabilizing or destabilizing. It may be tolerated smoothly in one context and poorly in another. The state itself does not provide the full explanation. The stability question is whether the system can enter, remain within, and leave that state without excessive disruption.

Glucose-dominant and fat-dominant states should be understood as relative shifts, not identities. The body does not use only glucose in one state and only fat in another. It shifts toward greater reliance on one fuel pattern or another depending on intake, demand, timing, signaling, and access. Careful language matters because absolute labels can turn regulatory states into categories they are not.

A more glucose-dominant condition often involves greater reliance on incoming or recently available fuel, glucose movement, insulin signaling, and post-intake distribution. This state can support function when access, uptake, conversion, and demand matching are coordinated. It can also become unstable if the movement of fuel is volatile, poorly timed, or mismatched to demand.

A more fat-dominant condition often involves greater reliance on stored fuel mobilization, sustained access, and internal reserves. This state can support continuity when mobilization and conversion are smooth. It can also become unstable if access is slow, demand is high, stress load is elevated, or recovery capacity is limited. Neither state is superior. Neither state is a moral category. Neither state guarantees stable energy. The important question is whether the system can move between states without producing instability.

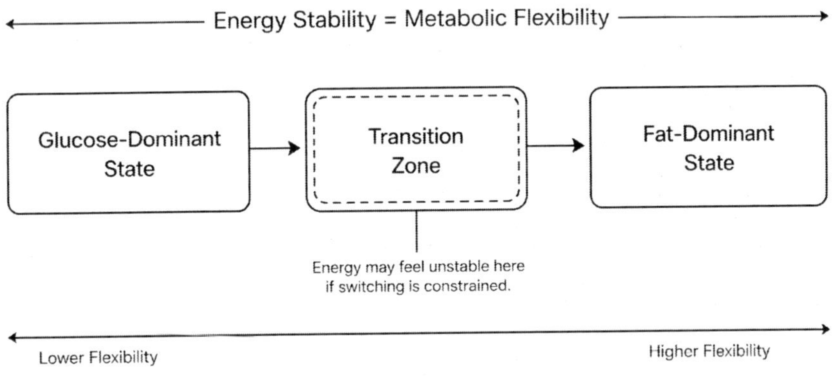

[Figure 7 — Fuel Transition Zone]

The transition zone is the core of this mechanism. It occurs when the system is moving from one fuel condition toward another. This can happen after meals, between meals, during longer gaps without intake, during increased activity, during stress, after `poor sleep, during long demand periods, when incoming fuel is becoming less dominant, when stored fuel access has not yet stabilized, or when stored fuel reliance is shifting back toward incoming fuel.

A transition zone is not automatically unstable. A smooth transition may include mild hunger, softening energy, changing alertness, or a lower-output window without breaking continuity. The system may shift fuel reliance while still preserving usable function. Energy may change, but the change remains tolerable and recoverable.

An unstable transition is different. It occurs when the system is moving away from one condition before the next condition is supporting output smoothly. The prior state is no longer carrying output in the same way, and the next state has not yet fully stabilized. This gap can be small and manageable, or it can become disruptive enough to appear as a dip, fog, urgency, heaviness, or reduced momentum.

This is why transition must be treated as its own mechanism rather than a brief bridge between fuel states. The instability may not belong to the fed state or the fasting state alone. It may belong to the movement between them. The strain may not mean glucose reliance is wrong or fat reliance is superior. It may mean the system is carrying a coordination load while shifting from one pattern of fuel use to another.

Transition burden is the coordination load created when the system has to shift fuel access, fuel conversion, appetite signals, glucose movement, insulin signaling, stress response, recovery state, and demand at the same time. During a transition, the person may experience one feeling, but the system may be coordinating many layers. The felt state compresses the burden into a single experience.

That experience may be hunger, fatigue, fog, urgency, heaviness, irritability, reduced momentum, or compensatory activation. These feelings are real, but they are not self-explanatory. The cost may come from the transition itself, not simply from lack of fuel. A person may feel hungry, but the pattern may also include glucose movement, appetite pressure, stress activation, and incomplete access to stored fuel. A person may feel foggy, but the system may be shifting fuel reliance while also carrying sleep debt or stress load.

This connects to the Perception Mechanism. The body translates internal conditions into felt energy, but the feeling does not identify every contributing layer. A transition can feel like a single energy problem while actually reflecting a layered coordination burden.

Switching tolerance is the system's ability to move between fuel states without excessive dips, urgency, fatigue, fog, hunger pressure, or compensatory strain. It is a system property, not a personal trait. It does not describe discipline, preference, or toughness. It describes how well fuel access, conversion, signaling, recovery, appetite pressure, and demand remain coordinated during state change.

Switching tolerance can be shaped by prior intake, fasting state, insulin signaling, glucose variability, metabolic flexibility, stress load, sleep state, recovery capacity, activity demand, appetite signaling, electrolyte balance, and fluid balance. These factors do not act independently. They define the condition of the system entering the transition. The same fuel transition may feel smooth under one condition and disruptive under another because the system receiving the transition has changed.

This variability explains why one transition cannot be interpreted in isolation. A gap between meals may feel ordinary on one day and destabilizing on another. Activity may be tolerated smoothly in one state and produce a dip in another. A post-meal shift may feel steady in one context and heavy in another. The transition is not only about the fuel state being entered. It is about the system's tolerance for the movement.

Switching range describes how many different fuel conditions the system can move through while preserving usable output. A wider switching range means the system can tolerate more variation in intake timing, demand, stress, and fuel reliance without repeatedly interrupting continuity. A narrower switching range means the system may function reasonably well in one condition but struggle when conditions shift.

Poor switching range does not mean fuel is absent. It means energy continuity depends too heavily on staying close to one condition. Energy may feel steady only shortly after eating. Urgency may appear quickly when incoming fuel is absent. Fog may appear during gaps between meals. Activity may produce disproportionate dips. Post-meal states may produce heaviness or volatility. Stress may make transitions sharper. Poor sleep may lower tolerance for fuel shifts.

A narrow switching range makes ordinary daily changes more disruptive. The system may not fail in a dramatic way, but it may lose continuity during common transitions. Moving from fed to between-meal state, from rest to activity, from low stress to higher demand, or from stored fuel reliance back toward incoming fuel may become costly. The issue is not that the body should avoid those transitions. The issue is that the range for smooth transition has narrowed.

Transition instability becomes visible as felt energy. Poorly tolerated transitions may feel like dips, urgency, hunger pressure, fatigue, fog, heaviness, irritability, reduced momentum, or compensatory activation. These are not diagnostic signs. They are possible ways state-change instability becomes experienced.

These experiences are often interpreted too narrowly. Urgency may be treated as simple hunger. Fog may be treated as random fatigue. Heaviness after eating may be treated as a property of the meal alone. Reduced momentum between meals may be treated as lack of effort. The Transition Mechanism offers a broader interpretation. These sensations may reflect the cost of moving between fuel states under the current regulatory conditions.

Stable energy requires fuel access, fuel conversion, and transition stability. If transitions are smooth, energy can change without breaking continuity. The system can move from incoming fuel toward stored fuel, from rest toward activity, from fasting toward feeding, or from lower demand toward higher demand without losing usable output.

If transitions are unstable, ordinary state changes become interruption points. This can contribute to crashes, drift, compensation, hunger-energy mismatch, post-meal instability, fasting instability, and activity-related dips. These later patterns do not all come from transition instability alone, but transition instability can be one layer beneath them.

The Transition Mechanism explains why energy can become unstable when the body shifts between fuel states, especially fed, fasting, more glucose-dominant, and more fat-dominant conditions. It includes dynamic fuel use, fed-state regulation, fasting-state regulation, relative fuel reliance, transition zones, transition burden, switching tolerance, switching range, and continuity impact. Energy instability can occur not because one fuel state is wrong, but because movement between states is poorly tolerated.

When transitions are smooth, energy can change state without becoming unstable. The system can shift, soften, mobilize, absorb, distribute, and recover while preserving continuity. But when a transition fails sharply, the result may not be a mild dip or gradual shift. Energy can fall quickly after a temporary rise, after a meal, after activation, or after apparent stability. That sharper pattern belongs to the next mechanism: the Crash Mechanism.

Crash Mechanism

Rapid energy decline after temporary elevation.

A crash often feels sudden. Energy may seem present, output may appear available, momentum may be holding, and then usable function drops quickly. The change may be felt as heaviness, fog, urgency, fatigue, reduced attention, lowered tolerance, irritability, or an abrupt need to stop. The shift can feel as if it arrived from nowhere because the moment of decline is the first moment when the system's instability becomes impossible to ignore.

At the surface, the crash looks like the beginning of the problem. Before it, function may have continued. The person may have been moving through demand, responding to pressure, completing tasks, staying alert, or relying on a temporary sense of momentum. Then output falls. Because the decline is experienced sharply, the crash appears to explain itself as a sudden event.

But a crash feels sudden because the drop is sudden, not necessarily because the cause began there. A crash feels sudden, but it is often built before it appears. The visible decline may be delayed evidence of instability that was already forming beneath the surface.

The crash is often the end of a chain. Earlier conditions may accumulate without immediately stopping output. Fuel access may be uneven. Glucose movement may be volatile. A transition between fuel states may be poorly tolerated. Stress activation may hold function in place temporarily. Sleep may have been insufficient. Recovery may be incomplete. Intake timing may be irregular. Demand may remain high. Output may continue through overextension, skipped recovery, illness load, or compensatory activation.

From a systems perspective, the crash is not random simply because it feels abrupt. It may represent the point at which the system can no longer preserve usable output under the conditions already created. The person notices the drop when function falls, but the system may have been moving toward that drop earlier through mismatched fuel access, rising strain, limited recovery, or unsupported elevation.

This timing gap matters. If the crash is treated only as the moment of decline, the earlier chain remains invisible. Attention goes to the low point, not the conditions that made the low point likely. The crash becomes interpreted as a failure of the moment rather than the visible endpoint of a longer pattern.

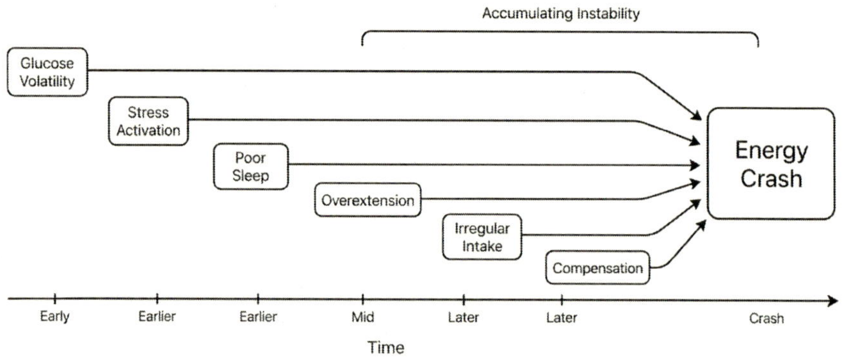

[Figure 8 — Crash as Delayed Output]

Temporary elevation is not stability. Energy may rise for many reasons. Incoming fuel may increase available substrate. Glucose movement may change felt alertness. Stress activation may create urgency or mobilization. A demanding environment may temporarily pull output upward. Task momentum may carry function for a period. Social pressure, internal pressure, stimulation, or compensatory output may allow the system to continue longer than its stable capacity would otherwise support.

None of these elevations is inherently good or bad. A temporary rise in output can be part of normal function. The issue is not elevation itself. The issue is whether continuity underneath is supported. A peak can hide fragility if the system does not have the fuel access, conversion tolerance, transition stability, and recovery capacity needed to sustain output after the elevation.

This returns the chapter to the book's central frame. Energy stability depends on continuity, not peaks. A period of high alertness does not prove that the energy system is stable. A productive window does not prove that output is supported. A burst of urgency does not prove that capacity is durable. The surrounding pattern determines whether elevation belongs to stability or compensation.

Elevation can be followed by decline when the rise is not supported by the rest of the system. Fuel access may not remain steady. Glucose movement may become volatile. The transition between fuel states may be poorly tolerated. Stress activation may fade. Demand may exceed conversion tolerance. Recovery capacity may be limited. The system may be borrowing from future capacity to maintain present output. Compensatory output may reach a limit.

One common pattern is that output rises first. The system appears to have energy available. Continuity underneath, however, is not fully supported. Cost accumulates while the person continues. Compensation holds output in place for a time. Then the compensation reaches its limit, and usable output drops. This is not the only crash sequence, but it illustrates why the crash can feel abrupt even when the instability was developing earlier.

Glucose volatility can be one contributor to this pattern. Rapid changes in available fuel or signal patterns may affect felt energy, especially when a rise is followed by a decline that the system does not buffer smoothly.

Post-intake regulation, glucose movement, insulin signaling, demand, and prior state can all shape whether energy feels steady or unstable.

But the Crash Mechanism is broader than glucose. Not every crash is a glucose crash. Not every post-meal decline has the same cause. Glucose volatility may be one layer in the chain, but crashes can also involve transition strain, poor sleep, stress activation, recovery limitation, illness load, irregular intake, high demand, and compensatory output. Reducing every crash to one fuel signal narrows the interpretation too quickly.

Stress activation adds another layer. Stress can create urgency, alertness, pressure, or mobilization that allows function to continue for a time. In that state, energy may feel available because activation is pushing output upward. But activation is not the same as stable energy. It may carry function temporarily while increasing the cost of maintaining that function.

Compensatory output is output maintained by extra strain rather than stable continuity. It is not a moral failure and not a virtue. It is a system pattern. The body may continue producing function by leaning on activation, urgency, pressure, or heightened mobilization when smoother support is limited. That output can appear effective while it lasts, but it may not be durable.

A crash may occur when compensatory output can no longer be maintained. The system may continue through demand for a period, then lose usable function rapidly once the supporting activation fades or the accumulated cost exceeds available recovery. The decline may feel like a sudden loss of energy, but the drop reflects the limit of a temporary support structure.

Recovery state shapes crash vulnerability. Poor sleep, under-recovery, illness load, accumulated strain, or high demand can reduce the system's ability to sustain output after elevation. Recovery state affects conversion tolerance because available fuel still has to become usable work. Recovery state also affects transition tolerance because moving between fuel states requires coordination. When recovery is limited, ordinary transitions can feel sharper and ordinary demand can become more expensive.

Demand load determines how quickly costs accumulate. A high-demand period can make temporary elevation more costly because output must remain elevated longer or more intensely than the system can support smoothly. Under-recovery can make ordinary output harder to sustain because the system begins the day with less available tolerance. The same elevation that would be manageable under one recovery state may be followed by a crash under another.

Irregular intake and transition strain can also contribute without becoming the whole explanation. Intake timing changes fuel access, appetite pressure, transition burden, and demand matching. The issue is not a rule about when food should appear. The issue is that timing changes the regulatory environment. If fuel-state transitions are already poorly tolerated, long gaps under demand or delayed access may make transitions sharper.

This connects directly to the Transition Mechanism. When the system is moving between fuel states, output may remain stable if the transition is smooth. But if the prior state is no longer carrying output in the same way and the next state has not stabilized, the transition can become costly. A crash may emerge when that poorly supported transition follows temporary elevation, delayed fuel access, stress activation, or accumulated demand.

The crash is not a moral failure. Crashes are often interpreted as laziness, lack of discipline, poor motivation, weakness, lack of seriousness, bad habits, or poor effort. Those interpretations confuse loss of usable output with character. A crash is a functional pattern under current conditions. It may involve fuel access, conversion tolerance, transition burden, recovery state, stress activation, and demand load.

Moving from blame to mechanism does not make the crash less real. It makes the crash more interpretable. The question becomes what conditions carried output before the drop, what supports were missing, what costs accumulated, and why continuity failed at that point. This is a more precise frame than treating the crash as a personal defect or a random interruption.

The Crash Mechanism connects directly to the Energy Continuity Mechanism. Stable energy means usable output can be sustained across time without excessive peaks, drops, or compensatory strain. A crash reveals a continuity failure. The problem is not always the low point itself. The pattern around the low point matters.

Crash analysis should look at the chain, not only the moment of decline. Was there a preceding elevation? Was output carried by activation? Was recovery limited? Was fuel access unstable? Was transition poorly tolerated? Was the system depending on compensation? Did output fall rapidly after appearing stable? These questions shift attention from the visible endpoint to the conditions that made the endpoint likely.

The Crash Mechanism explains rapid loss of usable output after temporary elevation, apparent stability, or compensatory activation. It includes temporary elevation, unstable fuel access, glucose volatility, transition strain, stress activation, compensatory output, recovery limitation, demand load, delayed system output, rapid decline, and continuity impact. A crash is not the beginning of instability. It is often the visible endpoint of instability that was built earlier.

Some energy instability appears as a sudden drop. Output holds, then falls. The change becomes obvious because the decline is sharp. But not all instability arrives in that form. Sometimes output does not crash. It slowly lowers. The baseline changes gradually enough that the shift may be easy to miss, and the system begins to operate from a reduced level of available function. That slower pattern belongs to the next mechanism: the Drift Mechanism.

Drift Mechanism

Gradual decline in baseline energy.

A crash announces itself through a sharp drop. Drift does not. A crash is noticed because usable output falls quickly enough to interrupt the day. Drift is slower, quieter, and easier to reinterpret as normal. It does not always arrive as a moment. It often appears as a gradual lowering of the level from which function begins.

A person may not notice drift when it starts. They may adjust expectations, reduce output, avoid certain demands, rely on more compensation, or accept lower energy as the new baseline. The change may not feel like instability at first because nothing has collapsed. The system continues operating, but from a slightly lower level. Over time, that lower level can become familiar.

Not all energy instability arrives suddenly; some instability becomes normal by lowering the baseline gradually.

Baseline energy is the ordinary level of usable function the system tends to return to across time. It is not a perfect number, a fixed trait, or a constant feeling. It is the general starting level from which demand, recovery, stress, feeding, fasting, movement, and sleep are experienced. Baseline energy is not the highest point of the day or the lowest point of a difficult moment. It is the functional ground the system repeatedly returns to.

This baseline matters because the same demand feels different depending on the starting point. A task that feels manageable from one baseline may feel expensive from another. A normal stressor may be absorbed when baseline function is higher and disruptive when baseline function has drifted downward. A meal, a fasting window, a period of activity, or a recovery window may all be experienced differently when the system begins from a reduced level of available output.

When baseline energy drifts downward, ordinary life can feel more expensive even before a dramatic crash occurs. The day may still be completed, but with less margin. Recovery may still happen, but more slowly. Demand may still be met, but with more strain. Drift changes the cost of normal function by lowering the starting point.

Drift happens gradually. Energy can decline over days, weeks, months, seasons, or longer periods. The movement may be too slow to notice day by day. There may be no single event that marks the change. Instead, the system adjusts in small increments until the new baseline feels familiar.

Tasks may require slightly more effort. Recovery may take slightly longer. Activity tolerance may narrow. Mornings may feel less restored. Stress may feel more costly. Gaps between meals may feel harder. Post-meal heaviness may appear more often. Attention may fade earlier. Compensatory patterns may become more common. None of these changes has to appear dramatic in isolation. Together, they can signal that the baseline has moved.

Drift often becomes visible only after the baseline has already shifted. The recognition may come when something that used to feel ordinary now feels costly, or when the person realizes that more of the day is organized around preserving output. The shift is delayed in awareness because the system adapts while the baseline is lowering.

Repeated conditions can shift the baseline. Drift is often built through recurrence rather than one extreme event. Poor sleep repeated over time, repeated stress, recovery debt, inconsistent fueling, illness or immune load, low movement tolerance, inactivity, overextension, chronic compensation, transition strain, or high demand without enough restoration can all contribute to a lower functional starting point.

The system may adapt to repeated conditions by lowering available output. This is not failure in a moral sense. It is a form of adjustment. If demand repeatedly exceeds restoration, the system may reduce the level of output it can make available without excessive strain. If stress activation repeatedly carries function, the system may begin operating with less margin. If transitions are repeatedly costly, tolerance may narrow.

The baseline does not shift because one difficult day occurs. It shifts when patterns repeat often enough that the system begins treating the lower level as the more sustainable operating point under current conditions. The body may conserve, reduce responsiveness, narrow tolerance, or increase the cost of additional demand. Drift is the visible energy consequence of repeated constraint.

This is why drift should not be interpreted as laziness, weakness, or permanent damage. It is a pattern of baseline movement under repeated conditions. The system is still regulating. It is still trying to preserve continuity. But it may be preserving continuity by lowering the amount of output it can reliably support.

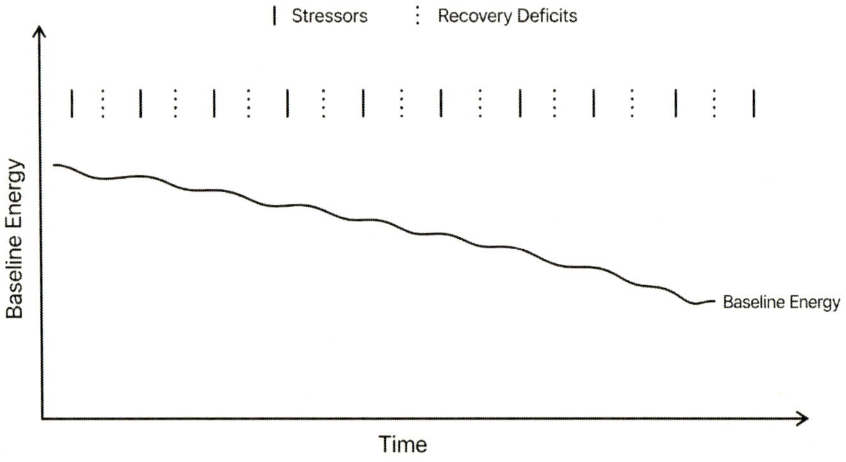

[Figure 9 — Baseline Drift]

Recovery mismatch is one of the central pathways into drift. Recovery mismatch occurs when the cost of output repeatedly exceeds the restoration that follows. It does not require one extreme event. It can accumulate through ordinary demand when the restoration after that demand is consistently incomplete.

Sleep, rest, lower demand, nutrition, illness recovery, and reduced strain all influence restoration capacity. These are not prescriptions in this chapter; they are system inputs. When restoration keeps pace with cost, baseline function has more support. When restoration repeatedly lags behind cost, the system may continue functioning but with less available margin.

Drift can occur when the system is not crashing sharply but is also not fully restoring. This is the quiet nature of drift. Output continues, but recovery does not fully return the system to its prior baseline. The next demand begins from a slightly lower level. Over time, those small reductions can accumulate into a new normal.

Stress load can also contribute to drift. Stress activation may temporarily preserve function by increasing readiness, urgency, or mobilization. In acute moments, that activation can help maintain output. But if activation becomes a frequent support layer, the system may begin operating at higher cost.

Chronic compensation means output is repeatedly maintained through extra strain rather than stable continuity. It differs from a single compensatory moment. It becomes a recurring pattern in which the system keeps function going by drawing on activation, pressure, urgency, or narrowed recovery margin. Function remains possible, but the cost of maintaining it rises.

The distinction between crash and drift is important here. A crash occurs when compensation reaches a limit sharply and output drops quickly. Drift occurs when compensation becomes routine and gradually lowers the baseline. Compensation can keep function going while quietly changing the level from which function begins. The system does not collapse, but it may become less available.

Inconsistent fueling and transition cost can also shape drift without reducing the chapter to eating rules. Inconsistent fueling matters because it may repeatedly change fuel access, appetite pressure, transition burden, and demand matching. The issue is not whether a single timing pattern is correct. The issue is how repeated fuel-state instability affects continuity.

If transitions are repeatedly sharp or poorly tolerated, the baseline may become less stable over time. The system may spend more energy adapting to shifts between incoming fuel and stored fuel, between fed and fasting states, or between lower and higher demand. Repeated transition burden can narrow tolerance, increase urgency, or make ordinary gaps feel more costly.

Drift may emerge when the system repeatedly spends energy adapting to unstable fuel-state changes. The cost does not always appear as a crash. It may appear as lower steadiness, less tolerance, more frequent heaviness, or a reduced sense of available output. Over time, the baseline adjusts around the repeated cost.

Movement tolerance adds another layer. Movement tolerance is the system's ability to handle physical demand without excessive cost or prolonged recovery. It is not a measure of virtue or identity. It is a capacity relationship between demand and recovery.

Both low movement exposure and overextension can contribute to drift in different ways. Inactivity may narrow tolerance because fewer demands are regularly supported, making ordinary movement feel more expensive. Overextension may exceed recovery capacity and increase accumulated strain. Low movement tolerance can make ordinary physical demand feel more costly, which may reduce the range of daily function the system can support comfortably.

Movement-related drift is therefore about tolerance and recovery matching, not moral judgment. A system exposed to too little demand may lose some tolerance for demand. A system exposed to too much demand without enough restoration may accumulate strain. In both cases, the baseline can shift downward because the relationship between output and recovery has become less stable.

Illness load and accumulated strain can also lower baseline energy. Illness, inflammation, immune activation, or ongoing physiological constraint can redirect resources, lower tolerance, increase recovery demand, and make baseline output feel reduced. This does not mean all persistent fatigue is metabolic or that every gradual decline has one explanation. It means that ongoing constraint can change the amount of output the system can make available.

Drift may reflect the system protecting or reallocating capacity under repeated constraint. When the system is dealing with illness load, inflammatory demand, or accumulated strain, lower output may represent an attempt to preserve function rather than a failure to generate it. The baseline shifts because the system is operating under a different set of demands.

The most difficult part of drift is normalization. Drift hides by becoming familiar. A lower baseline can begin to feel normal because the comparison point has changed. The person may stop noticing how much function has narrowed because the narrowed range becomes the new reference point.

Expectations may adjust. Higher-demand activities may be avoided. Compensatory routines may become part of the day's structure. The lowered state may be interpreted as personality, age, laziness, busyness, or inevitability. The person may not think of energy as declining because the decline has been absorbed into daily assumptions.

The point is not to deny aging, life demands, or real constraints. Those factors matter. The point is that slow baseline movement can become difficult to see once it is familiar. Drift does not need to announce itself as instability. It can become the background condition from which everything else is interpreted.

This connects directly to the Energy Continuity Mechanism. Stable energy is not only about avoiding crashes. It also requires protecting the baseline from gradual erosion. A system can avoid dramatic drops while still losing continuity if the starting point steadily lowers.

A lower baseline changes tolerance for demand, recovery after effort, transition stability, appetite-energy alignment, stress resilience, conversion tolerance, and the likelihood of crashes. When the starting point is lower, ordinary variation has less room to occur before it becomes disruptive. Dips feel larger. Transitions feel sharper. Recovery takes longer. Stress consumes more of the available range.

Drift weakens continuity by lowering the starting point and narrowing the range of tolerable variation. The system may still function, but with less margin. Stability becomes more fragile because less disruption is required to create a noticeable decline.

The Drift Mechanism explains gradual downward movement in baseline energy when repeated conditions make lower functional output more likely, more familiar, or more tolerable to the system. It includes gradual decline, baseline shift, delayed recognition, recovery mismatch, stress load, chronic compensation, inconsistent fueling, transition cost, movement tolerance, illness load, accumulated strain, normalization, and continuity erosion. Drift is not a moral failure. It is adaptation under repeated conditions.

Drift shows how instability can become quieter over time. The system may not collapse, but it may begin operating from a lower baseline. One reason drift can persist is that compensation often keeps function going long enough for the shift to feel normal. The next chapter turns to that compensation directly: the short-term supports that preserve output while increasing future instability.

Compensation Mechanism

Short-term boosts that mask underlying instability.

Instability does not always stop function immediately. A person may continue moving, responding, deciding, eating, engaging, working, or meeting obligations while the system is already under strain. Output may remain visible even while the internal cost of that output is rising. The day may still proceed, but the support structure underneath it may be changing.

This makes instability difficult to see. When function continues, the surface signal appears reassuring. The person is still present, still responding, still completing ordinary demands. But visible function is not the same as stable function. A system can maintain output for a period while relying on support mechanisms that increase strain, narrow tolerance, or delay the cost until later.

Continued output is not always the same as stable output. Stable output is supported by continuity. It can persist without excessive peaks, sharp drops, baseline erosion, or repeated compensatory strain. Compensated output also persists, but it persists through added support. The distinction is not visible only in the moment. It becomes clearer through what the output costs, how recovery follows, and whether the same support has to be used repeatedly.

Compensation can preserve function temporarily while hiding the instability that made compensation necessary.

Compensation is the use of short-term supports to preserve function when ordinary continuity is not fully supported. It is not failure. It is not automatically harmful. It is not a character defect. It is a preservation strategy. The body compensates because it is designed to adapt to changing demand. Behavior compensates because daily conditions often require function even when internal support is imperfect. Environments can also support compensation by reducing choices, narrowing demands, or supplying external structure.

The important distinction is between stable support and compensatory support. Stable output is carried by coordinated fuel access, conversion, transition tolerance, recovery capacity, and demand matching. Compensatory output is carried by extra strain. It may rely on activation, urgency, narrowed attention, momentum, habit, stimulation, social demand, or forced continuation.

This does not mean compensation should never happen. A system that could not compensate would be fragile. Temporary supports are part of ordinary adaptation. The question is not whether compensation occurs. The question is whether compensation is absorbed through recovery or repeated until it changes the system.

Body-based compensation can make energy feel available even when continuity is not fully stable. Stress activation may increase alertness or readiness. Mobilization may make output possible for a period. Urgency may sharpen response. Attention may narrow so fewer competing signals interfere with the immediate demand. Fatigue perception may be temporarily delayed.

These shifts can be useful in the short term. Narrowed attention, for example, can preserve output by reducing the field of demand. The system focuses on what must be handled now, while other signals become less prominent. This can make function feel clearer, sharper, or more available, but it does not prove that the underlying system has more stable capacity. It may simply mean that the system has changed signal priority.

Fatigue perception can also be delayed without the underlying cost disappearing. The body may continue output by suppressing or postponing the felt signal of strain. Appetite pressure or sleep pressure may shift afterward because the system still has to account for the cost that was temporarily hidden. The person may feel capable during the compensatory window, then experience stronger hunger, difficulty settling, heaviness, or fatigue later.

Activation can create usable output without proving that continuity is stable. This is one reason compensation is easy to misread. The system may feel more capable in the short term precisely because it is calling on a higher-cost support layer.

Compensation can also be behavioral and environmental. Momentum can carry a person through a sequence after readiness has already declined. Habit can reduce decision demand by allowing familiar actions to continue without requiring repeated evaluation. External deadlines and social pressure can organize output temporarily by narrowing attention around what must be completed. Structured routines can preserve function because they reduce variability.

Reduced choices can also function as compensation. When the system has less range available, narrowing the day can preserve output. Fewer options mean fewer transitions, fewer decisions, and fewer demands on flexibility. Avoiding higher-demand tasks, shortening the day's range of activity, or relying on easier patterns may make the system appear stable because the visible output remains intact.

This does not make those patterns wrong. They may be practical short-term supports. The mechanism matters because compensation can be hidden inside routines that appear functional from the outside. The person may seem stable because the environment has been shaped to require less variability, less transition, and less recovery flexibility.

Because compensation keeps output going, it can create the impression that the system is fine. Output can be mistaken for capacity. Completing the day can be mistaken for having moved through the day with continuity. Maintaining a routine can be mistaken for energy stability.

But output can continue while continuity is deteriorating. Compensation can precede a crash when it holds function in place until the support reaches a limit. It can also allow drift to feel normal when repeated supports keep daily function moving while the baseline gradually lowers. In both patterns, compensation delays recognition because function has not stopped yet.

The core cycle begins when continuity is not fully supported. Fuel access, conversion tolerance, transition stability, recovery capacity, or demand matching may be incomplete. Instead of output stopping immediately, compensation preserves function. The person continues. The task is completed. The day proceeds.

While output continues, cost accumulates. The cost may not appear in the same moment because compensation postpones the signal. It may be carried into appetite, sleep, irritability, fatigue, recovery delay, or lower next-day output. The system has maintained function, but maintaining function required something extra.

Future strain increases unless recovery follows. Repeated compensation can increase dependence on compensation because the system begins to rely on the same support layers to meet ordinary demand. Tolerance can narrow. Transitions can become sharper. Movement can feel more costly. Stress sensitivity can rise. The baseline may lower gradually because restoration never fully catches up with the cost of maintained output.

The problem is not compensation itself. The problem is repeated compensation without restoration. Compensation is destabilizing when it becomes the substitute for continuity rather than a temporary bridge back to it.

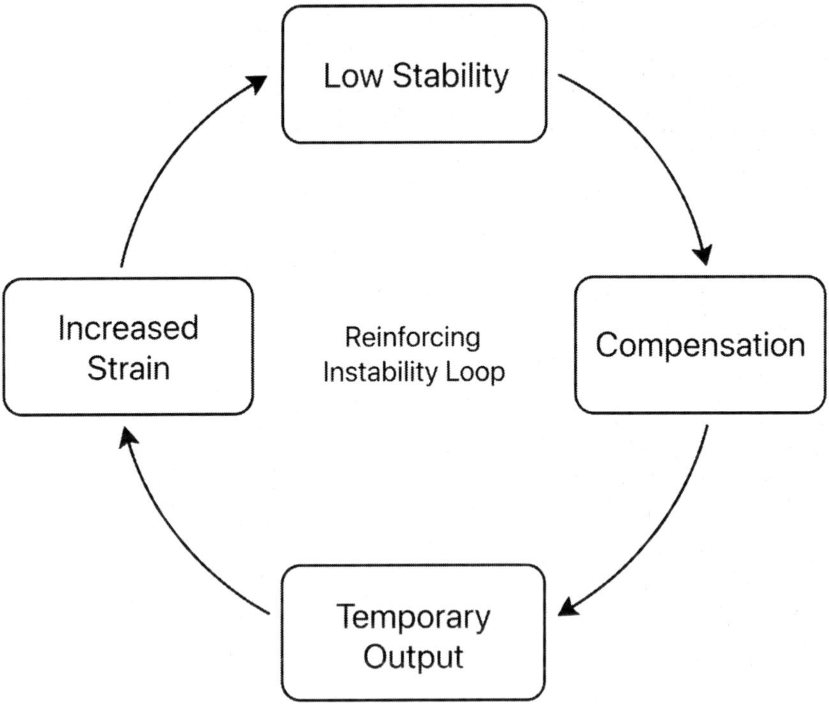

[Figure 10 — Compensation Cycle]

Recovery determines the meaning of compensation. Temporary support can be absorbed when the system has enough restoration afterward. Life sometimes requires higher demand, unusual timing, stress, illness, travel, family needs, work pressure, or disruption. In those contexts, compensation may preserve function until conditions change.

Compensation without recovery becomes different. It can become a repeated operating mode. Acute compensation may contribute to crashes when the support fails sharply. Chronic compensation may contribute to drift when output continues but the baseline gradually lowers. Repeated compensation raises future cost because the system has fewer opportunities to restore the continuity that compensation replaced.

Compensation must be interpreted by what happens next. A short-term support followed by restoration has a different meaning than the same support repeated daily without recalibration. The mechanism is not defined only by the support itself. It is defined by repetition, cost, and recovery.

The cost of compensation may appear later, and it may appear somewhere else. Output maintained by activation may appear later as difficulty settling down or altered sleep pressure. Output maintained by urgency may appear later as irritability, reduced patience, stronger hunger, cravings, or appetite pressure. Output maintained by narrowed routines may appear later as reduced range. Output maintained by stimulation may appear later as lower baseline or stronger dependence on stimulation.

This is cost migration. The system preserves output in one place, and the cost becomes visible in another. A demanding period may not produce an immediate crash, but it may alter appetite signals later. A day carried by urgency may be followed by heavier fatigue. A routine that preserves function by narrowing activity may reduce tolerance for broader demand.

This connection reaches into appetite without making appetite the whole explanation. Hunger, cravings, and urgency can reflect more than preference or behavior. They may appear as downstream signals after output has been maintained at higher cost. The cost of compensation may appear in a different system than the one that preserved output.

Compensation can also contribute to baseline drift. If compensation repeats often enough, it can become routine. The system may begin treating compensatory output as the normal way to function. More output requires more activation. Ordinary demand feels more expensive. Recovery no longer fully restores baseline. Lower output becomes familiar.

Compensation can hide the lower baseline because function continues. The person is still moving through the day, but with more support required to produce the same visible output. Over time, the system may preserve the day while slowly changing the level from which the next day begins.

This is why compensation can become difficult to identify once it becomes routine. The support layer stops feeling like a temporary adjustment and begins to feel like part of ordinary function. More activation, more narrowing, more external structure, or more recovery delay may be treated as normal because the visible output has not disappeared. The system is still producing function, but the conditions required to produce that function have become more expensive.

In this sense, compensation does not only protect the current day. It can also shape the next day's starting point. When the cost of preserved output is not restored, the following baseline may begin with less margin, less tolerance, and greater dependence on the same compensatory supports. The pattern reinforces itself because the lower baseline makes compensation more likely, and repeated compensation makes full restoration harder to reach.

Compensation is not the enemy. Life requires temporary supports. The body is designed to compensate. Behavior often has to compensate. A system that can preserve function under imperfect conditions has adaptive capacity.

The issue is not that compensation occurs. The issue is whether compensation becomes the default substitute for stable continuity. The goal is interpretation, not elimination. Compensation becomes meaningful when it reveals the difference between output that is supported and output that is merely maintained.

Stable energy means usable output can be maintained across time without excessive peaks, crashes, drift, or compensatory strain. Compensation sits at the boundary between stability and instability. It may preserve continuity briefly, but it may also increase future instability if repeated without recovery.

This is why compensation explains how energy instability can remain hidden while output continues. It reveals the difference between output being present and continuity being supported. The system may still be functioning, but the cost of that function may be accumulating beneath the surface.

The Compensation Mechanism explains how short-term supports preserve usable output under unstable conditions while potentially increasing future strain if recovery, restoration, or recalibration does not follow. It includes temporary preservation, instability masking, body-based compensation, behavioral compensation, environmental compensation, stress activation, urgency, momentum, habit, stimulation, forced output, delayed cost, cost migration, recovery dependence, future strain, and continuity impact. Compensation is not failure. It is a short-term preservation strategy whose meaning depends on repetition, cost, and recovery.

This hiddenness matters because the next section of the book turns toward system interactions. The system may still be functioning, but the support structure underneath may be changing. One of the most visible signals involved in these shifts is glucose: not because glucose explains every energy pattern, but because glucose movement can shape alertness, urgency, dips, post-meal changes, and perceived availability. The next chapter turns to that interaction directly.

Glucose Interaction Mechanism

Blood sugar variability and energy fluctuations.

Glucose is easy to over-read because it is measurable, visible, and closely associated with energy. When energy rises or falls, glucose can appear to be the obvious explanation. A dip may feel like blood sugar. Post-meal heaviness may be attributed to blood sugar. Hunger, irritability, fog, urgency, and fatigue may all be interpreted through glucose alone because glucose is one of the clearest signals people have learned to associate with fuel availability.

That attention is understandable. Glucose is not abstract. It changes across time, responds to food, shifts with activity and stress, interacts with insulin, and can influence how available energy feels. It is connected to fuel access and signal coordination. When energy feels unstable, glucose is one of the first patterns that can seem relevant.

But glucose becomes misleading when it is treated as the whole explanation. Energy is not produced by glucose alone. Stable daily function also depends on insulin signaling, fuel access, conversion, transition tolerance, appetite signals, sleep state, stress load, recovery capacity, activity demand, electrolyte and fluid balance, and the broader system context in which glucose movement occurs. Glucose is one important energy signal, not the whole energy system.

Glucose can be understood as one fuel-availability signal. Its movement can influence perceived energy because it reflects part of the system's available fuel pattern. Changes in glucose can affect alertness, urgency, post-meal state, hunger pressure, and the felt sense that output is available or becoming less available. In this way, glucose belongs directly inside the Energy Stability framework.

But glucose presence is not the same as usable energy. Chapter 4 established that fuel must become accessible, coordinated, and matched to demand. Chapter 5 showed that accessible fuel must still be converted into usable functional output. Chapter 6 added that the system must tolerate transitions between fuel states. Glucose participates in each of these layers, but it does not replace them.

A glucose pattern may show that fuel is moving through the system, but that fuel still has to be distributed, taken up, converted, and integrated with current demand. If recovery is limited, stress load is high, insulin coordination is strained, or transition tolerance is narrow, glucose availability may not translate cleanly into stable energy. Glucose availability is not the same as energy continuity.

Stable glucose patterns can support smoother perceived energy by reducing one layer of volatility. When glucose movement is less abrupt and better coordinated with demand, the system may have fewer sharp dips to buffer. Alertness may feel steadier. Hunger or urgency signals may be less abrupt. Post-meal states may feel less disruptive. Transitions between incoming fuel and stored fuel may be easier to tolerate.

This does not mean stable glucose guarantees stable energy. It means that one signal layer is less volatile. The rest of the system still matters. Insulin signaling must coordinate distribution. Fuel must be converted into work. Sleep and recovery must support tolerance. Stress load must not dominate the signal environment. Demand must remain within a range the system can meet.

Stable glucose can support smoother energy, but it does not carry the whole system alone. A person can have less glucose volatility and still feel low energy if recovery is poor, stress load is high, illness load is present, or conversion tolerance is reduced. Glucose stability is supportive, not totalizing.

Volatile glucose patterns can contribute to energy instability when movement is rapid, poorly buffered, or poorly matched to demand. A sharp rise and decline may be felt as fluctuating availability. A dip may contribute to hunger, urgency, fatigue, irritability, fog, reduced attention, or a sense that function is suddenly less accessible. The felt experience may be sharper when glucose movement interacts with stress, appetite pressure, or transition strain.

This connects to crashes without making every crash a glucose event. Glucose volatility may be one layer in rapid energy decline, especially when a temporary rise is followed by a poorly tolerated drop. It also connects to compensation. When energy feels unstable, the system may lean on urgency, activation, narrowed attention, or other short-term supports to preserve function while fuel and signals stabilize.

Glucose volatility can contribute to energy instability without being the only cause of it. A crash-like experience may involve glucose movement, but it may also involve poor sleep, high stress, limited recovery, transition burden, inconsistent fuel access, or compensatory strain. The value of glucose is that it provides one visible signal. The risk is mistaking that signal for the entire system.

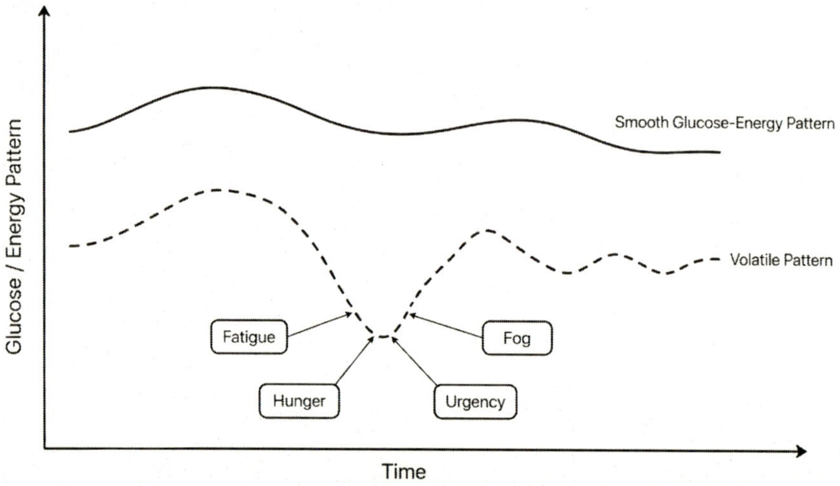

Glucose variability can shape perceived energy.
It is one pathway among many that influence overall energy stability.

[Figure 11 — Glucose Variability and Energy]

Post-meal energy is one of the most common places glucose is over-interpreted. A person may feel steady after eating in one context and heavy, foggy, or unstable in another. The immediate interpretation may be that the meal itself explains the entire energy response, or that glucose alone explains the whole post-meal state. Both interpretations are incomplete.

Post-meal energy reflects the meal interacting with the system receiving it. Meal composition can matter because different inputs change digestion, glucose movement, insulin signaling, and appetite resolution in different ways. Timing can matter because the same intake may land differently depending on current demand, prior intake, or the length of the preceding gap. Prior state can matter because the body receiving the meal may be rested, stressed, under-recovered, already activated, or carrying accumulated strain.

Insulin response matters because glucose movement is coordinated rather than simply present. Sleep state matters because poor sleep can alter perceived energy, appetite signaling, stress reactivity, and fuel handling.

Stress load matters because stress can change urgency, activation, and regulatory priorities. Activity and demand matter because fuel that arrives during low demand may feel different from fuel that arrives before, during, or after higher demand.

Recovery state and transition tolerance also shape post-meal energy. If recovery is limited, digestion and fuel distribution may occur inside a system with less tolerance for additional load. If transition tolerance is narrow, the shift from fasting or between-meal state into a fed state may feel more disruptive. The same meal may therefore produce different energy experiences because the system context has changed.

A glucose dip may also be felt through several different signals. It may be interpreted as fatigue, hunger, urgency, irritability, fog, reduced attention, shakiness, need for immediate intake, or reduced tolerance. These sensations are real, but they are not self-explanatory. The body translates internal changes into felt experience, and glucose movement may be one of the signals involved.

This connects directly to the Perception Mechanism. A felt dip does not automatically identify its origin. The same glucose movement may feel mild in one context and disruptive in another. Stress can amplify urgency. Poor sleep can make the same change feel heavier. Appetite pressure can make a dip feel more urgent. Limited recovery can reduce the system's ability to buffer the signal.

A glucose dip may shape felt energy, but the feeling does not identify glucose as the only layer. Not every hunger signal is a glucose dip. Not every fatigue signal is glucose-related. Not every moment of fog is caused by blood sugar movement. Glucose can participate in the felt state without owning the entire explanation.

Glucose also interacts with appetite. Changes in glucose may contribute to hunger pressure, cravings, urgency, or the sense that intake is needed soon. This connection matters because appetite is one of the ways energy instability becomes behaviorally visible. When perceived availability drops, appetite signals may intensify.

But appetite is not explained by glucose alone. Appetite signals are shaped by insulin, stress, sleep, prior intake, recovery state, habit, environment, compensation, and learned timing patterns. Hunger and cravings may include a glucose component, but they may also reflect recovery debt, stress activation, sleep disruption, or prior restriction. Glucose can influence appetite signals without explaining appetite by itself.

Glucose variability can also increase compensation pressure. When glucose movement feels unstable, the system may rely more heavily on activation, urgency, stimulation, or narrowed routines to preserve output. A dip may invite compensatory activation. Post-meal heaviness may encourage forced output or a reduced range of activity. Hunger urgency may increase the pressure to respond quickly.

Compensation may preserve function while glucose and other signals stabilize. This can make the glucose-energy relationship harder to interpret. Output may continue, but not because the system is stable. It may continue because compensation has temporarily covered the instability. Over time, repeated compensation can blur the relationship between glucose movement, felt energy, and actual continuity.

Glucose must therefore be interpreted in broader system context. Insulin signaling determines how fuel is routed, stored, accessed, and distributed. Appetite signals shape urgency and eating response. Sleep affects glucose handling, stress reactivity, recovery tolerance, and perceived readiness. Stress can alter both glucose movement and the felt meaning of that movement.

Activity changes demand and fuel use. Recovery determines whether available fuel can be converted into usable output without excessive strain. Electrolyte and fluid balance influence circulation, signaling, and physical ease. Fuel transitions shape whether the system is moving smoothly between incoming and stored fuel reliance. Conversion tolerance determines whether available fuel becomes functional output. Demand load determines how much support is required.

The same glucose movement can therefore feel different in different contexts. A modest dip may be barely noticed when sleep, stress, recovery, and demand are well aligned. A similar dip may feel urgent when stress is high, appetite pressure is elevated, or recovery is limited. A post-meal rise may feel stabilizing in one condition and heavy in another because the system receiving that rise is not the same.

The meaning of glucose movement depends on the system state around it. Energy continuity depends on coordination across systems, not on glucose alone. Glucose is important because it is visible, responsive, and closely tied to fuel availability. It is incomplete because energy stability requires the interaction of fuel, signaling, conversion, recovery, demand, and perception across time.

The Glucose Interaction Mechanism explains how blood sugar variability interacts with energy continuity by influencing perceived fuel availability, alertness, dips, hunger, urgency, post-meal energy, and crash risk within the broader context of insulin signaling, appetite, stress, sleep, recovery, activity, and transition tolerance. It includes glucose as signal, perceived fuel availability, stable patterns, volatile patterns, dips, post-meal energy, hunger, urgency, irritability, fog, crash risk, compensation pressure, system context, and continuity impact.

Glucose is one important energy signal, not the whole energy system. Its patterns can support continuity or contribute to instability, but only inside a broader regulatory field. The question is not whether glucose matters. It does. The question is how glucose interacts with the other layers that determine whether daily energy remains usable, recoverable, and stable across time.

Glucose movement helps explain part of energy variability, but glucose does not act alone. Every glucose pattern is interpreted through coordination: where fuel is moving, what is being stored, what is being used, what is being accessed, and how the system directs energy across tissues and time. That coordination brings the next signal into view: insulin. The next chapter turns to insulin not as a villain or a force, but as an energy distribution signal.

Insulin Interaction Mechanism

Energy distribution and storage signals.

Insulin is often framed as either the enemy or the entire explanation for metabolic instability. In one version of the misreading, insulin is treated as a problem by itself. In another, it becomes the master key that explains every change in energy, appetite, storage, fatigue, or body composition. Both frames are too narrow. Insulin matters, but it matters because it coordinates where energy goes. Coordination is not the same as blame.

The distortion happens because insulin sits close to visible metabolic outcomes. It responds after intake. It interacts with glucose. It influences storage and access. It changes across fed and fasting states. Because these effects are visible and meaningful, insulin can easily become moralized. Higher insulin may be treated as failure. Lower insulin may be treated as virtue. That framing removes insulin from its actual role inside regulation.

Insulin is not good or bad; it is a routing signal that shapes energy distribution and access. This distinction is essential for Energy Stability because daily energy depends not only on whether fuel appears, but on where that fuel is directed, how accessible it remains, and whether routing matches current demand.

Insulin helps the body handle nutrients after intake and across metabolic states. It influences how fuel is moved, stored, accessed, and used. Chapter 10 described glucose as a visible fuel signal. Glucose movement shows part of the fuel-availability pattern. Insulin helps coordinate what happens to that fuel. It shapes whether fuel remains circulating, moves into tissues, enters storage, becomes available for use, or becomes less accessible under current conditions.

This is why insulin should not be reduced to a storage hormone in a narrow sense. Storage is one route, but it is not the whole signal. Insulin participates in distribution. It helps coordinate movement between circulation, tissue uptake, storage, and later access. Storage itself is not failure. It is one way the system preserves future availability and maintains continuity across time.

Insulin does not merely store energy; it coordinates energy routing. That routing matters because energy stability depends on matching supply with need. A system that cannot route fuel well may have fuel present while still experiencing unstable output. A system that routes fuel smoothly can support continuity by directing energy where it is needed, storing what is not immediately required, and shaping access across changing conditions.

After intake, nutrients enter the system and must be handled. Food does not arrive as stable functional energy. It enters a regulatory environment. Glucose movement requires coordination. Amino acids, fatty acids, and other nutrients must be distributed. Different tissues have different needs at different times. Some fuel may be used soon. Some may be stored. Some may remain circulating briefly while the system adjusts.

Insulin helps coordinate this post-intake distribution. It supports movement into tissues where fuel can be used or stored. It helps organize the transition from incoming fuel management toward later access. This process is not separate from energy stability. The way fuel is handled after arrival influences post-meal energy, later dips, appetite signals, transition tolerance, and perceived availability.

Post-intake energy is therefore not only about fuel arriving. It is about how fuel is routed after arrival. A meal may introduce fuel, but insulin signaling helps determine how that fuel is distributed. If routing and demand align smoothly, energy may feel steadier. If routing and demand are mismatched, fuel may be present while usable output feels reduced, heavy, urgent, or unstable.

The central routing outcomes are circulation, use, storage, and restricted access. Circulation means fuel remains available in the bloodstream for a period. This can support access, but circulation alone does not guarantee stable output. Fuel still has to reach the tissues that need it, be taken up, and be converted into work.

Use means fuel is taken up and converted into functional output. This route supports real-time energy when access, conversion, oxygen delivery, recovery state, and demand are coordinated. It is the route most directly connected to felt output, but it still depends on the broader system.

Storage means fuel is moved into reserve. This is a normal system function. Storage preserves future availability and helps prevent the system from needing all incoming fuel to be used immediately. In a stability frame, storage is not moral failure. It is one route within energy regulation.

Restricted access means some fuel may become less accessible under current conditions. This does not mean the fuel has disappeared. It means the signaling state may favor other routes, such as storage or circulation management, while limiting access to certain reserves. Restricted access can affect perceived energy even when stored energy exists because stored fuel is not automatically usable fuel.

None of these routes is inherently good or bad. Each can support or disrupt energy continuity depending on timing and demand. Circulation can support availability or contribute to volatility. Use can support output or exceed recovery capacity. Storage can preserve future access or feel mismatched when immediate demand is high. Restricted access can be appropriate in one state and destabilizing in another. Energy depends not only on how much fuel exists, but on where that fuel is routed and how accessible it remains.

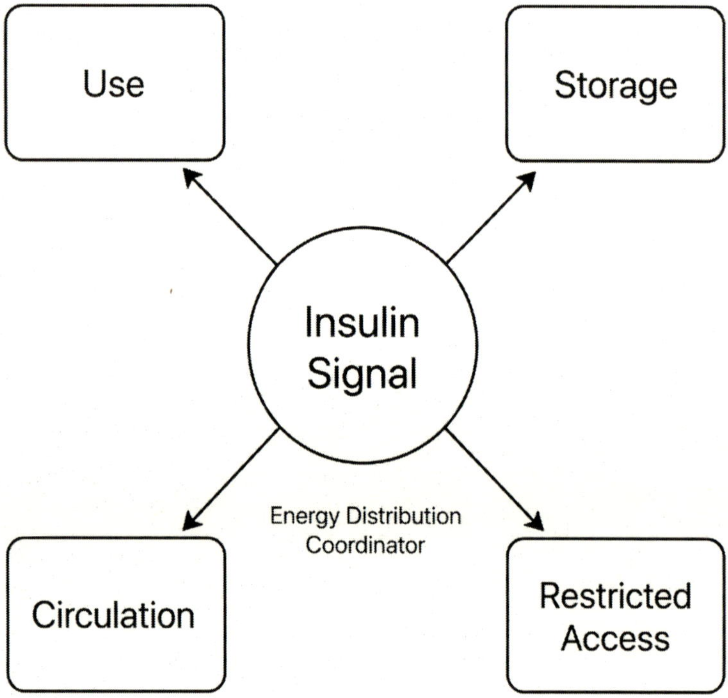

[Figure 12 — Insulin as Energy Distribution Signal]

Energy instability can emerge when fuel routing and current demand are poorly matched. Demand may require available fuel while routing moves more fuel toward storage. Circulating fuel may change before tissues have the access needed for stable output. Access to stored fuel may be reduced under current signaling conditions. Recovery state or stress state may alter the demand side of the equation. Activity may increase fuel needs before routing has adjusted.

This mismatch can be felt as reduced energy, urgency, heaviness, fatigue, or the need for compensation. The issue is not that insulin is wrong. The issue is that distribution and demand are not aligned smoothly enough to preserve continuity. Fuel exists, but the pattern of routing does not match the pattern of need.

Insulin tone describes the signal environment around fuel routing. Higher or more prolonged insulin tone can create different access patterns than lower-insulin states. This does not mean higher insulin is automatically bad or lower insulin is automatically better. It means the system is operating under different routing conditions.

Higher or more prolonged insulin tone may favor storage and reduce access to certain stored fuels under current conditions. Lower insulin states may allow different access patterns, including greater reliance on mobilized reserves. Both states can be appropriate depending on context. After intake, routing incoming fuel is necessary. During longer gaps without intake, access to stored fuel may become more relevant.

Problems arise when insulin state, demand, recovery, and transition tolerance are mismatched. A lower-insulin state does not guarantee stable energy if transition tolerance is poor or recovery capacity is limited. A higher-insulin state does not automatically produce instability if distribution and demand are coordinated. Different insulin states create different access patterns; no state is automatically virtuous.

Glucose and insulin should be interpreted together. Glucose movement creates coordination demand. Insulin helps coordinate that movement. A glucose rise is not just a fuel event; it is a routing event. The system has to decide how much fuel remains circulating, how much is used, how much enters storage, and how access changes afterward.

Glucose changes may feel different depending on insulin response. A post-meal glucose pattern may feel steady in one context and heavy or unstable in another because insulin signaling, demand, recovery state, and stress load differ. Insulin response may shape post-meal energy, later dips, storage, access, and transition into the next fuel state.

Glucose is the visible fuel signal; insulin shapes how that signal is handled. This pairing prevents glucose from being interpreted alone and prevents insulin from being treated as a separate moral force. The interaction matters because energy continuity depends on coordinated movement, not isolated measurements.

Insulin can also interact with appetite and energy perception. It may influence whether fuel feels available, resolved, or restricted. It can shape the post-meal state, the timing of hunger return, the sense of satisfaction, or the urgency that appears when routing and demand do not align. These effects matter because appetite is one way internal energy state becomes behaviorally relevant.

But appetite is not insulin alone. Energy perception is not insulin alone. Hunger, cravings, urgency, satiety, and readiness are shaped by glucose movement, stress load, sleep state, prior intake, recovery, habit, environment, and compensation. Insulin can shape appetite and energy perception without explaining either by itself.

Storage and fat access must be interpreted neutrally. Storage is a normal system function. Fat storage is not moral failure. It is one way the body preserves energy availability across time. Stored fuel supports the system by creating reserves that can be accessed later under appropriate conditions.

At the same time, stored fuel is not the same as accessible fuel. Chapter 4 established this distinction directly. Energy may exist in storage while not feeling available in the moment. Access from storage depends on state, demand, signaling, transition tolerance, and metabolic context. Insulin state can influence access to stored fuel by shaping whether the system is oriented more toward storage, circulation management, or mobilization.

This matters for energy continuity because reserves do not automatically solve real-time output. Stored energy supports the system, but stored energy is not automatically available energy. The question is whether signaling, access, demand, and conversion are aligned enough for reserves to support function when needed.

Fasting transitions add another layer. As insulin tone changes, fuel access patterns can change. Fed and fasting states involve different routing conditions. In the fed state, incoming fuel is being managed, distributed, and stored where appropriate. In fasting states, the system relies more on internal reserves, mobilization, and adjusted access patterns.

Lower insulin states may allow more stored-fuel access, but that does not mean they always feel better. Transition tolerance matters. If the system shifts poorly between fed and fasting states, the change in insulin tone may be felt as fatigue, urgency, fog, or compensatory activation. Smooth transitions support continuity because fuel access changes without repeatedly interrupting output.

Insulin must be interpreted in broader system context. Glucose movement, appetite signals, sleep, stress, activity, recovery, electrolyte and fluid balance, fuel transitions, fat storage, demand load, and energy perception all shape what insulin signaling means in practice. Identical insulin states may feel different under different conditions because the system around the signal is different.

A post-intake insulin response after good recovery and moderate demand may support stable distribution. A similar response under poor sleep, high stress, or narrow transition tolerance may feel different. Insulin matters because routing matters. It is incomplete because routing is only one layer of energy stability.

The meaning of insulin signaling depends on the system state around it. Energy continuity depends on coordination across systems: fuel must appear, be routed, be accessed, be converted, and be matched to demand while recovery and stress load shape tolerance. Insulin is central to routing, but daily energy is larger than routing alone.

The Insulin Interaction Mechanism explains how insulin signaling influences energy continuity by routing nutrients toward use, storage, circulation, or restricted access, shaping whether available fuel becomes usable output, stored reserve, or less accessible under current demand. It includes insulin as coordination signal, nutrient routing, post-intake distribution, circulation, use, storage, restricted access, distribution-demand matching, insulin tone, glucose interaction, appetite interaction, energy perception, fasting transitions, storage access, system context, and continuity impact.

Insulin is not good or bad. It is a routing signal that shapes energy distribution and access. Its importance comes from its role in coordination, not from any moral quality. Energy instability becomes clearer when insulin is understood as part of the system that determines where fuel goes, when it becomes available, and whether routing matches demand.

Insulin helps explain how energy is routed, stored, used, and made more or less accessible. But energy continuity is not only a matter of internal routing. The body also has to translate energy state into behavior. Hunger, satiety, cravings, urgency, and eating response become the interface between internal energy conditions and daily action. That brings the next mechanism into view: appetite as the behavioral interface of energy stability.

Appetite Interaction Mechanism

Hunger and energy misalignment.

Appetite is easy to interpret as a direct reading of energy need. Hunger may be treated as proof that energy is absent. Cravings may be treated as weakness or desire. Muted appetite may be treated as control or stability. Satiety loss may be treated as lack of discipline. These interpretations are incomplete because appetite feels immediate, but immediacy does not make a signal fully explanatory.

Appetite is often moralized because it sits close to behavior. Hunger leads toward eating. Cravings narrow attention. Satiety affects stopping. Muted appetite can be interpreted as restraint. Because appetite signals are felt and acted upon, they are easily confused with character, choice, or self-control. That framing removes appetite from the system that produces it.

Energy and appetite are closely connected, but they do not perfectly reveal each other. Energy state can influence hunger, cravings, satiety, and urgency. Appetite can also shape future energy through eating response. But appetite is not a direct meter of available energy, and energy is not a simple reflection of appetite. Appetite and energy are connected, but they are not identical.

Appetite is the behavioral interface between internal energy state and eating response. It translates internal conditions into pressure, urgency, quietness, or resolution. It is not simply "wanting food." It includes hunger, cravings, satiety, fullness, muted appetite, urgency, and loss of resolution. These signals help move internal state toward behavior, but they are shaped by many layers before they appear.

Glucose movement, insulin signaling, stress load, sleep state, recovery capacity, prior intake, habit, environment, and compensation all influence appetite. A hunger signal may reflect fuel availability, but it may also reflect routine timing, stress state, or prior restriction. A craving may reflect urgency, learned response, glucose movement, fatigue, or compensation. A loss of satiety may reflect incomplete energy resolution rather than a failure of restraint.

Appetite is where internal energy conditions become behaviorally visible. This matters for Energy Stability because appetite can either support continuity or reveal misalignment. When appetite signals align reasonably with energy need and response, eating behavior may help preserve function. When they misalign, the system may experience urgency, delayed response, cravings, fatigue, or later instability.

Hunger is often a forecasting signal, not only a report of immediate absence. Hunger may rise when the system detects falling availability, anticipates future demand, senses routine timing, or responds to prior conditions. It can appear before output fails because the system is not waiting for complete depletion before signaling need.

This changes the interpretation of hunger. Hunger can reflect current fuel state, but it can also reflect predicted need. A person may feel hunger before a demanding period, during a familiar meal window, after a stretch of unstable glucose movement, or when prior intake did not produce durable resolution. The signal is real, but it is not always a direct measurement of current energy deficit.

Hunger often forecasts energy need before energy continuity actually fails. That forecasting role can support stability when the signal appears in proportion to need. It can become destabilizing when the forecast is amplified, delayed, muted, or poorly matched to actual demand. The question is not whether hunger is valid. The question is what system state it is forecasting.

Cravings narrow attention around expected relief. They are not automatically weakness or failure. A craving can focus the system toward a specific response, often one associated with fast access, learned resolution, familiarity, or prior relief. The specificity of a craving does not make it moral. It suggests that the system has learned a particular pathway from discomfort toward resolution.

Cravings may be shaped by glucose movement, stress, sleep loss, habit, prior restriction, environment, and compensation. They can appear when the system seeks fast resolution or when appetite pressure becomes narrowed around a known response. A craving may therefore reflect urgency, not character.

This does not mean cravings always identify the best response or a precise physiological need. It means they are signals of narrowed attention. They show how appetite can compress many internal conditions into a focused behavioral pull. Cravings narrow attention around expected relief, not simply desire.

The central misalignment in this chapter involves three layers: energy need, hunger signal, and eating response. These layers can align, but they can also fall out of sync. Energy need may be present while hunger is muted. Hunger may be high while stored energy is abundant. Eating response may not match the actual need. Appetite signals may lag behind energy state, overshoot, or undershoot.

Prior conditions can distort the signal. Poor sleep can alter hunger and cravings without reflecting only immediate fuel need. Stress can suppress appetite temporarily and then increase urgency later. Compensation can mask energy need until the system has already accumulated cost. Glucose and insulin dynamics can influence perceived availability without explaining appetite alone.

Eating response adds another layer. The response may come early, late, strongly, weakly, narrowly, or inconsistently. It may be shaped by environment, habit, access, routine, learned timing, or stress. Energy need, hunger signal, and eating response do not always move together.

When these layers fall out of sync, continuity can be affected. Misalignment may contribute to fatigue, urgency, overeating, under-eating, cravings, or later crashes. The issue is not moral failure. It is a signal-response mismatch. Energy need, hunger signal, and eating response can fall out of sync.

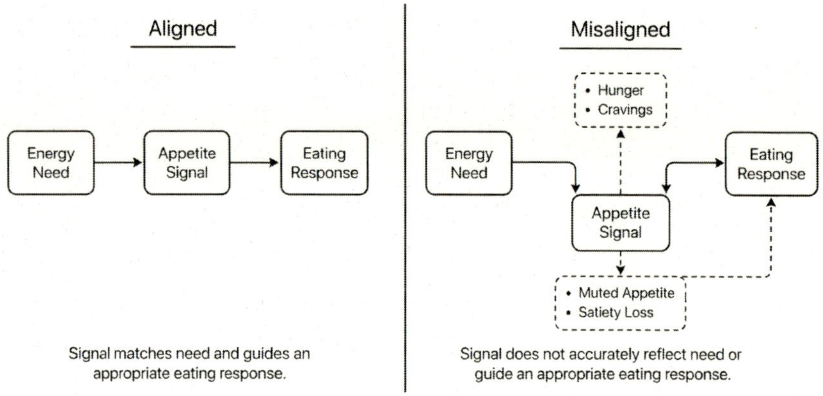

[Figure 13 — Appetite-Energy Misalignment]

Muted appetite is also easily misread. It may be interpreted as control, discipline, or stability. In some contexts, muted appetite can reflect genuine resolution after adequate intake or a stable post-meal state. Appetite quietness is not inherently a problem.

But low appetite does not automatically mean energy stability. Appetite can become muted during stress activation, illness, compensation, fatigue, disrupted signals, or reduced awareness. The system may suppress eating pressure while still carrying high energy cost. A person may feel low output and low appetite at the same time.

Muted appetite can also delay eating response until later urgency appears. When appetite quietness reflects activation rather than resolution, the signal may return sharply once the activation fades. The important distinction is that muted appetite can mean different things depending on context. Low appetite does not automatically mean energy stability.

Satiety loss creates another form of misalignment. Satiety is not simply fullness. Fullness describes a physical sense of volume or immediate post-meal presence. Satiety describes the durability of post-meal resolution. It is the length and stability of the period in which appetite pressure settles and perceived energy feels supported.

Satiety loss occurs when that resolution fades sooner than expected or does not hold. It can shorten the interval of stable perceived energy and precede hunger, cravings, urgency, dips, or compensation. A person may have eaten, but the energy-appetite system does not remain resolved long enough to preserve continuity.

Satiety loss can reflect meal-system mismatch, glucose and insulin dynamics, stress load, sleep state, prior restriction, recovery debt, or transition strain. It is not a discipline problem and does not require a food rule to interpret. Satiety loss can be an early signal that energy resolution is not holding.

Appetite can also feel high when stored energy is abundant because stored energy is not automatically accessible energy. Chapter 4 established that stored fuel is not the same as available fuel. Chapter 11 showed that insulin signaling can influence access, routing, storage, and distribution. Appetite responds to perceived availability, forecasted need, and signal state, not merely the existence of reserves.

Stored energy does not automatically quiet appetite. If accessible fuel feels limited, if the system forecasts demand, if transition tolerance is narrow, or if stress and sleep disrupt signals, appetite may rise even when reserves exist. High appetite does not prove lack of stored fuel. It reflects the system's interpretation of availability and need.

The opposite misalignment also occurs. Energy can feel low even when appetite is quiet. Stress activation may suppress appetite while increasing energy cost. Illness or fatigue may reduce appetite while output remains low. Compensation may delay appetite signals. Poor sleep may alter hunger and energy separately.

Low appetite can coexist with low output because appetite is one interface, not the entire energy system. The system may have limited recovery, reduced conversion tolerance, high stress load, or illness-related constraint while appetite remains muted. Energy can be low even when appetite is quiet.

Appetite-energy misalignment can increase compensation pressure. Hunger urgency may pull attention toward immediate response. Cravings may narrow attention around expected relief. Muted appetite may delay response until later strain. Satiety loss may increase repeated pressure to respond. In each case, appetite signals can shape behavior in ways that affect future energy.

Compensation may also hide appetite-energy mismatch until later. A person may continue through urgency, fatigue, or muted appetite using activation, routine, or external demand. Later cost may appear as hunger rebound, irritability, fatigue, cravings, or lower baseline. Appetite misalignment can become compensation pressure when the system uses short-term support to keep functioning despite unresolved signal mismatch.

Appetite must be interpreted in broader system context. Glucose movement can influence urgency and perceived availability. Insulin signaling can affect routing and post-meal resolution. Sleep changes appetite pressure, stress reactivity, glucose handling, and recovery. Stress can suppress appetite temporarily or amplify urgency later. Recovery state affects how costly demand feels and how strongly appetite signals appear.

Activity, electrolyte and fluid balance, meal timing, prior intake, habit, environment, compensation, and energy perception all shape appetite. Identical hunger can mean different things in different contexts. Identical energy states can produce different appetite signals depending on sleep, stress, prior intake, and recovery. Appetite is meaningful, but its meaning depends on the system state around it.

Energy continuity depends on appetite signals being reasonably aligned with actual need and response. Appetite matters because it influences future energy through eating behavior. It can support continuity when it helps match intake, demand, and recovery. It can disrupt continuity when signals become amplified, muted, delayed, or misread.

The Appetite Interaction Mechanism explains how hunger, cravings, muted appetite, and satiety loss interact with energy continuity by translating internal fuel state, forecasted need, signal instability, prior conditions, and perceived availability into eating pressure or eating suppression. It includes appetite as behavioral interface, hunger forecasting, cravings and attention narrowing, muted appetite, satiety loss, energy need, hunger signal, eating response, stored versus accessible energy, low energy with low appetite, high appetite with stored energy available, compensation pressure, system context, and continuity impact.

Appetite and energy are connected, but they are not identical. Appetite is one way internal energy conditions become behaviorally visible, but it must be interpreted through glucose, insulin, sleep, stress, recovery, environment, habit, and compensation. It is a signal interface, not a moral test and not a complete explanation.

Appetite helps translate energy state into behavior, but the accuracy and durability of that translation depend heavily on recovery state. Sleep changes glucose handling, appetite pressure, stress reactivity, recovery capacity, and perceived readiness. When sleep is constrained, appetite-energy alignment becomes harder to maintain. The next chapter turns to sleep as one of the core constraints shaping energy stability.

Sleep Constraint Mechanism

Recovery capacity and energy restoration

Sleep is often treated as a simple tiredness variable. More sleep is assumed to reduce tiredness. Less sleep is assumed to increase it. Within that framing, sleep becomes a quantity problem, and energy becomes a feeling that rises or falls in proportion to that quantity. This interpretation is understandable because tiredness is the most immediate and visible consequence of sleep disruption. It is what can be felt first.

But tiredness is not the full effect of sleep. Sleep does not merely change whether a person feels tired. It changes the system that produces next-day energy. The distinction is not semantic. It shifts sleep from a surface-level sensation into a structural input. When sleep is reduced, it is not only tiredness that changes. The capacity to generate stable output the following day changes as well.

Sleep influences next-day capacity, signal tolerance, and energy volatility. A poorly restored system does not simply feel more tired. It begins the day from a different baseline. Signals that would otherwise be absorbed smoothly may feel sharper. Ordinary demand may carry greater cost. Variability may increase. Sleep is not just rest; it is system restoration for next-day energy capacity.

Sleep functions as a restoration layer. It supports repair, rhythm, nervous system recovery, metabolic regulation, signal recalibration, and recovery capacity. These processes are not experienced directly as discrete events, but their effects are expressed through how the system behaves the next day. Energy stability depends on the integrity of these layers.

Repair is one aspect of this restoration. Tissue-level processes, cellular maintenance, and broader system upkeep are supported during sleep. This does not translate into a simple "recharged" feeling. It influences whether the system begins the next day with enough structural support to handle demand without accumulating strain.

Rhythm is another aspect. Sleep contributes to the alignment of timing signals across systems. Hormonal patterns, metabolic readiness, and neural coordination follow rhythms that are shaped by sleep. When rhythm is disrupted, signals may still occur, but their timing and coordination may become less stable. This affects how energy is produced and maintained across the day.

Nervous system recovery is also central. Sleep allows the system to reset from prior activation. Without sufficient restoration, the system may begin the next day closer to a state of strain. This does not require extreme conditions. It can appear as increased reactivity, reduced tolerance for interruption, or faster escalation of effort under ordinary demand.

Metabolic regulation is influenced as well. Sleep affects how glucose is handled, how appetite signals are generated, and how fuel is accessed and used. These changes do not require a large shift in intake to be felt. The same intake can produce different perceived outcomes depending on how restored the system is.

Sleep restores the system that energy has to come from. Energy is not produced in isolation. It emerges from a coordinated system that depends on prior restoration. When restoration is reduced, energy output may still occur, but it may require more effort, show greater variability, or rely more heavily on compensation.

The next day does not begin from neutral. It begins from the recovery state left by the prior night. This establishes sleep as a baseline setter. The system does not reset to zero between days. It carries forward the condition produced by prior restoration.

When sleep supports restoration, the system may begin with more margin. Margin refers to the capacity to absorb ordinary demand without immediately approaching instability. With more margin, transitions may feel smoother, signals may be less amplified, and output may be sustained with less perceived cost.

When restoration is incomplete, the starting point shifts. Baseline energy may be lower. This does not necessarily mean a person cannot function. It means the same level of function may require more effort or produce more strain. Ordinary tasks may feel heavier not because they have changed, but because the system absorbing them has less available capacity.

This connects to the Drift Mechanism. Repeated nights of incomplete restoration can gradually lower the baseline from which the system operates. The change may not be immediately obvious because function can continue. But over time, lower baseline becomes more familiar, and higher baseline may feel less accessible.

Sleep shapes the baseline from which energy continuity begins. It determines whether the system starts with margin or with accumulated strain.

Sleep debt can be understood as an accumulated restoration gap. It does not require an extreme deficit to have an effect. Even modest reductions in restoration, when repeated, can alter how the system behaves. The effect is not only a lower baseline but also increased variability.

With reduced restoration, energy may become less stable across the day. Dips may appear more quickly. Irritability may increase. Appetite pressure may become less predictable. Stress sensitivity may rise. Compensation may be required earlier or more frequently to maintain output.

Transitions may feel sharper. Moving from one task to another, from rest to activity, or from one level of demand to another may require more adjustment. This can increase the perceived cost of change, even when the absolute demand is not high.

Crashes may become more likely when demand exceeds restored capacity. This does not mean that every period of reduced sleep leads to a crash. It means that the margin for absorbing demand is reduced, so the threshold for instability is reached more easily.

When repeated, reduced restoration can contribute to drift. Lower baseline and increased variability can become normalized. The system may begin to operate in a narrower range, with greater reliance on compensation to maintain continuity.

Poor restoration can create both lower baseline and greater volatility.

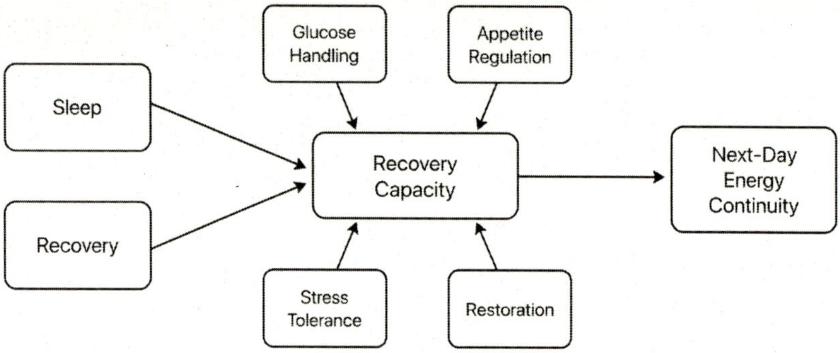

[Figure 14 — Sleep as Recovery Input]

Sleep state also influences how glucose is handled and experienced. After reduced restoration, glucose patterns may feel more volatile even when intake is similar. The same meal can produce a different perceived energy response depending on how restored the system is.

Post-meal energy may become less predictable. Heaviness, dips, or urgency may feel sharper. This does not require large changes in glucose values. It reflects how the system interprets and manages those values under different restoration conditions.

The distinction is not that sleep directly changes glucose in a single direction. It changes how glucose movement is handled and felt. A well-restored system may buffer variability more smoothly. A poorly restored system may experience the same variability as more disruptive.

Sleep state changes how glucose movement is handled and felt.

Appetite signals are also affected. Reduced restoration may increase appetite pressure, shorten satiety durability, or increase cravings and urgency. Timing may shift, with hunger appearing earlier, later, or more unpredictably.

Satiety may fade more quickly. A meal that would normally produce a sustained period of resolution may produce a shorter interval before hunger or urgency returns. This does not require a change in meal composition to be experienced. It reflects how the system processes and integrates the intake under different conditions.

Cravings may become more specific or more frequent. This can reflect the system seeking faster resolution under conditions of reduced stability. Again, this is not a moral problem. It is a change in signal behavior.

Sleep state changes how appetite signals are generated and interpreted.

Sleep also affects stress tolerance. The system's ability to absorb ordinary demand depends on how restored it is. With reduced restoration, the same demands may feel more activating. The threshold for strain may be lower.

The nervous system may begin closer to a state of activation. This can appear as increased urgency, irritability, or reactivity. Minor disruptions may feel larger. Tasks that require sustained attention may feel more effortful. This is not a change in the tasks themselves. It is a change in the system processing them.

Reduced stress tolerance can increase compensation pressure. The system may rely more on activation, routine, or external structure to maintain output. This can preserve function in the short term but increase future strain if restoration does not follow.

Poor restoration reduces the margin available for ordinary demand.

Recovery capacity describes the system's ability to absorb demand without becoming unstable. It is not the same as motivation. It is not a measure of willingness or effort. It is a measure of available restoration margin.

With higher recovery capacity, ordinary demand can be absorbed with less cost. Tasks can be completed with less perceived strain. Transitions can occur more smoothly. Signals may remain within a range that supports continuity.

With lower recovery capacity, the same demand produces more strain. Tasks feel heavier. Transitions require more adjustment. Signals may amplify more quickly. Compensation may be required sooner to maintain output.

This is why the same task can feel different on different days. The task has not changed. The recovery capacity absorbing it has changed. A level of demand that is manageable with sufficient restoration may feel costly when restoration is reduced.

Recovery capacity determines how much ordinary demand the system can absorb before output becomes unstable.

Energy continuity depends on several underlying layers. Repair supports structural integrity. Rhythm supports timing and coordination. Nervous system recovery supports readiness without excessive activation. Metabolic regulation supports glucose handling, appetite signaling, and fuel access.

These layers are not separate from energy. They are the conditions from which energy emerges. When they are restored, energy output can be sustained with less volatility. When they are disrupted, energy may become more variable, more costly, or more dependent on compensation.

Feeling rested is one expression of restoration, but it is not the full picture. A person may feel temporarily alert after reduced sleep, especially if compensation is engaged, but still have reduced recovery capacity. The system's underlying state determines continuity more than momentary perception.

Energy continuity depends on restored regulation, not only on feeling rested.

The effects of reduced restoration often appear the next day rather than during the night itself. Sleep changes the system that must produce output. The consequences are expressed when that system is used.

The next day may begin with a lower baseline. Energy may feel reduced from the start, or it may decline more quickly once demand begins. Dips may appear earlier. Transitions may feel more difficult. Signals may amplify more quickly.

Appetite pressure may increase. Cravings may become more prominent. Irritability or urgency may appear under ordinary conditions. Compensation may be used to maintain output, increasing future strain.

This delayed effect explains why energy instability often appears the day after reduced restoration. The night does not contain the instability. It shapes the system that produces it.

Energy instability often appears the day after poor restoration because sleep changes the system that must produce output.

Sleep should not be treated as a moral test. It is a constraint layer. Sleep can be influenced by work demands, caregiving, stress, illness, environment, schedule instability, pain, or life conditions. These factors are not always controllable, and they do not reflect character.

Poor sleep is not a failure. It is a condition that alters the system's capacity. The purpose of understanding this mechanism is not to assign blame. It is to interpret why energy may feel different under different restoration states.

Sleep matters, but it does not explain every energy problem. Energy stability depends on multiple interacting layers. Sleep is one of them. Its influence can be significant, but it is not exclusive.

Sleep is a constraint layer, not a character judgment.

The Sleep Constraint Mechanism explains how sleep affects energy continuity by restoring recovery capacity, regulatory rhythm, nervous system readiness, metabolic coordination, and tolerance for next-day demand. It includes sleep as a restoration layer, next-day baseline, sleep debt, energy volatility, glucose handling, appetite pressure, stress tolerance, recovery capacity, repair, rhythm, nervous system recovery, metabolic regulation, demand absorption, delayed instability, and continuity impact.

Sleep is not just rest. It is system restoration for next-day energy capacity. It determines how the system begins, how it responds, and how it sustains output across the day.

Sleep restores the system's capacity to absorb demand, but demand itself also matters. Even a restored system has limits when readiness demands, emotional load, cognitive demand, illness pressure, uncertainty, or environmental strain accumulate. The next chapter turns to stress not as a psychological label alone, but as a load state that can redirect energy, alter signals, and constrain durable output.

Stress Load Mechanism

How readiness demands disrupt durable energy continuity.

Stress is often treated as a psychological state, an emotional complaint, or a mindset problem. Under that framing, stress appears to belong mainly to thought, mood, or interpretation. This is understandable because stress is often felt through attention, tension, irritability, pressure, worry, or urgency. These are the parts of stress most available to awareness.

But stress is not only psychological. It is also a readiness demand. It changes how the body allocates attention, fuel, signal priority, output, and recovery bandwidth. Stress prepares the system to respond, and that preparation affects energy. It can raise alertness while increasing cost. It can make output feel available while reducing durability. It can help the system meet immediate demand while making continuity harder to preserve.

Temporary activation is not the same as durable energy capacity.

Stress is a whole-system readiness state. It changes system priorities. Instead of organizing primarily around restoration, digestion, steady signaling, or long-range continuity, the system may shift toward response. Attention becomes more selective. Fuel may be mobilized differently. Appetite signals may change. Glucose patterns may become more reactive. Sleep pressure may be altered. Fatigue perception may be pushed into the background.

This does not make stress inherently bad. A readiness state can be useful. The body needs ways to respond to demand, uncertainty, threat, urgency, and increased load. Stress becomes relevant to energy stability because readiness is not free. When the system organizes around response, other processes may receive less bandwidth.

Stress is therefore a load state that changes readiness, not merely a feeling. It can preserve function temporarily while changing the cost of that function. The person may experience the state as focus, pressure, urgency, or alertness, but beneath that experience the system is reorganizing priorities.

This explains why stress can feel like energy. Stress activation may increase alertness, urgency, focus, speed, and output. Readiness can make action feel more available. Urgency can sharpen attention by narrowing the field to what must be handled now. Activation can temporarily suppress fatigue perception, allowing output to continue even when restoration is incomplete.

This temporary increase can be useful. A system that could not mobilize under demand would be fragile. The problem is not that activation occurs. The problem is interpreting activation as proof of durable capacity. Stress can raise output temporarily without increasing the system's underlying ability to sustain output across time.

Temporary alertness is not the same as restored capacity. Activation increases readiness. Durable energy requires recovery capacity, fuel access, conversion, regulation, and tolerance. A person can feel alert while the system is not restored. A person can continue producing output while baseline energy is eroding. A person can appear functional while compensation is carrying the difference.

Activation can hide fatigue until later. It may push fatigue perception out of awareness, but it does not erase the cost of output. This connects directly to the Compensation Mechanism. Stress activation can preserve function when ordinary continuity is not fully supported. It can make the system feel capable in the short window while increasing future strain.

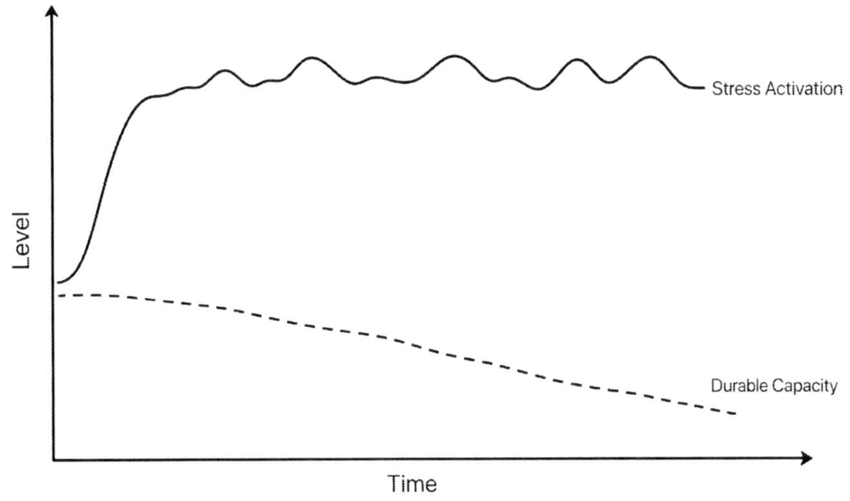

Wired and depleted can occur at the same time.

[Figure 15 — Stress Activation vs Durable Capacity]

Sustained stress increases system cost. The system cannot remain in heightened readiness without some consequence. Readiness requires fuel, attention, signal coordination, regulatory adjustment, and recovery tradeoffs. When activation is brief and followed by restoration, the cost may be absorbed. When activation is sustained or repeated, the cost becomes part of the energy pattern.

Output maintained under stress may feel urgent or available, but it may carry higher cost than output supported by stable continuity. The same task performed under high readiness may consume more recovery bandwidth. The same conversation, decision, or demand may feel more expensive. The system is not only doing the task. It is doing the task while maintaining a heightened readiness state.

The cost may appear later. Fatigue may arrive after the activating demand ends. Irritability may increase as tolerance narrows. Appetite pressure may shift because the system has carried additional load. Sleep may become less restorative if activation continues into the recovery window. A crash may follow when compensatory activation can no longer hold output in place.

Repeated stress load can also contribute to drift. The system may keep functioning, but from a gradually lower baseline. More output may require more activation. Ordinary demand may feel more costly. Recovery may no longer fully restore the prior starting point. The same stress response that supports short-term function can disrupt long-term continuity.

Recovery bandwidth is the capacity available for restoration while the system is also responding to demand. Under lower stress load, more bandwidth may be available for repair, digestion, appetite resolution, nervous system recovery, and baseline restoration. Under higher stress load, the system may remain oriented toward output even when rest time exists.

This explains why time away from demand does not always feel restorative. If readiness remains elevated, the system may have less bandwidth for restoration. Stress may make it harder to settle. It may shorten recovery windows by keeping attention and physiology oriented toward response. It may carry cost into sleep and next-day baseline.

Stress load can reduce the bandwidth available for restoration. The issue is not merely how much time is available. It is how much of the system can shift from readiness into recovery. When that shift is incomplete, energy continuity becomes more vulnerable the next day.

Stress and sleep reinforce each other. Poor sleep reduces stress tolerance, leaving the system with less margin for ordinary demand. Stress load can make restoration less complete by keeping readiness high. Activation can interfere with settling, and incomplete restoration can make the system more reactive the following day.

This loop can increase volatility over time. A poorly restored system may respond more strongly to ordinary stress. Higher stress may then reduce restoration further. Energy may become more variable, not because one signal has failed, but because readiness and restoration are falling out of sync.

Stress also changes the context in which glucose and insulin signals are handled. Stress can alter glucose patterns and perceived availability by changing the demand side of fuel regulation. The system may require more immediate readiness, and glucose movement may feel sharper or more urgent under that condition.

Insulin signaling also occurs inside the stress state, not apart from it. A similar glucose or insulin pattern may feel different when readiness is high because demand, appetite, recovery, and perception are different. Stress changes the system interpreting the signal. The same fuel pattern may feel stable in one state and strained in another.

Stress can distort appetite-energy alignment in either direction. Appetite may become muted during acute activation because signal priority shifts toward immediate response. Hunger may return later with more urgency once activation fades. Cravings may narrow attention around expected relief. Satiety may feel less durable. Timing may become less predictable.

This does not mean stress explains appetite by itself. Appetite remains shaped by glucose, insulin, sleep, recovery, prior intake, habit, environment, and compensation. Stress matters because it changes signal priority. It can suppress, amplify, delay, or sharpen appetite signals depending on the broader system state.

Wired energy is one of the clearest expressions of the Stress Load Mechanism. A person can feel alert and depleted at the same time because activation and restoration are different layers. The system may be highly ready while also under-recovered. It may be difficult to settle even while baseline energy is low.

Wired energy is not proof of stable energy. It is activation layered over depletion. High readiness can coexist with low recovery capacity. Fatigue perception may be suppressed while cost accumulates. The body can remain activated even when it does not have durable capacity underneath that activation.

This explains why the person may feel unable to stop while also feeling exhausted. The system remains oriented toward response. Attention stays narrowed. Signals remain amplified. Yet the underlying restoration margin is limited. The result is not true continuity. It is readiness without sufficient recovery.

This distinction matters because wired energy can be misread from both directions. From the outside, it may look like high function because output is still present. From the inside, it may feel confusing because the body seems activated but not restored. The person may be moving, thinking, responding, or completing tasks, yet the underlying state does not feel settled or durable. The signal is mixed because the system is carrying two conditions at once: readiness remains elevated, while recovery capacity remains limited.

In that state, stopping may not feel easy even when continuing is costly. The system may remain organized around response, making rest feel unavailable despite exhaustion. This is one reason stress load can blur the line between energy and activation. The presence of motion, alertness, or urgency does not prove that the system has stable energy underneath. It may only show that the readiness layer is still dominant.

Stress load increases energy volatility by raising output cost and reducing recovery margin. Energy may rise temporarily and then drop. Dips may become sharper. Baseline may become less predictable. Compensation may be used more frequently. Appetite and sleep disruption may add additional instability.

Over time, stress load can contribute to crash, drift, and compensation patterns. It can support temporary output before a crash. It can maintain function while baseline slowly lowers. It can require repeated compensation to keep output going. Stress is not the only cause of these patterns, but it can make each of them more likely by increasing cost and reducing restoration.

Stress is a constraint, not a character judgment. Stress can come from work, caregiving, uncertainty, illness, pain, financial pressure, conflict, environmental demand, cognitive load, emotional load, or schedule instability. These are not simply mindset problems. They are conditions that place readiness demands on the system.

Stress response is adaptive. The issue is not whether stress exists. A living system must respond to demand. The issue is whether readiness demand repeatedly exceeds restoration capacity. When that happens, energy continuity becomes harder to preserve.

The Stress Load Mechanism explains how readiness demands affect energy continuity by increasing activation, redirecting signal priority, raising short-term output, increasing system cost, reducing recovery bandwidth, and making energy more volatile when activation is sustained or repeated without restoration. It includes stress as readiness demand, whole-system activation, temporary alertness, fatigue suppression, signal priority, output cost, recovery bandwidth, sleep interaction, glucose interaction, insulin context, appetite distortion, wired exhaustion, energy volatility, crash risk, drift risk, compensation pressure, and continuity impact.

Temporary activation is not the same as durable energy capacity. Stress can support function in the short term, but energy stability depends on whether output remains usable, recoverable, and sustainable across time without excessive compensatory strain.

Stress load shows how readiness demand can redirect energy, alter signals, and increase the cost of maintaining output. But durable energy also depends on the physical conditions that allow signals, circulation, nerve activity, and muscle function to remain coordinated. The next chapter turns to electrolytes and fluid balance not as hydration accessories, but as constraints on signal integrity and fatigue perception.

Electrolyte Constraint Mechanism

Signal integrity and fatigue perception.

Electrolytes are often treated either as hydration accessories or quick fixes for fatigue. In one frame, they are reduced to something added to water. In another, they are treated as if they directly produce energy. Both frames are incomplete because they turn an infrastructure layer into a shortcut. Electrolytes matter, but not because they act like fuel, stimulation, or a direct source of output.

This misreading is understandable. Electrolyte and fluid balance can be felt physically. Changes in tolerance, heaviness, dizziness, weakness, or physical ease can feel immediate, and immediate sensations invite simple explanations. If the body feels heavy or unstable, it is easy to look for a single missing input. If electrolyte language is framed around quick relief, the mechanism becomes compressed into a correction story.

But electrolyte and fluid balance are not best understood as quick correction tools. They are part of the physical infrastructure that allows energy to be expressed. Energy requires communication, circulation, nerve signaling, muscle function, pressure tolerance, and fluid stability. Electrolytes support these conditions. They do not create energy by themselves.

Electrolytes do not create energy; they support the signaling and fluid conditions that allow energy to be expressed.

Energy must be expressed, not merely produced. Fuel availability is not enough. Conversion is not enough. A system may have fuel present and still experience weak, heavy, dizzy, poorly coordinated, or low-tolerance output if the physical expression layer is strained. Energy becomes useful only when it can move through the body as coordinated function.

This links directly back to fuel availability and energy conversion. Chapter 4 asked whether fuel could become reachable. Chapter 5 asked whether reachable fuel could become usable work. Chapter 15 adds another layer: whether usable work can be expressed through tissues, circulation, nerves, muscles, posture, movement, pressure tolerance, and coordinated action.

Energy is felt through action. Standing requires coordination. Walking requires repeated signaling. Posture requires sustained muscular tone. Attention depends on circulation, nervous system regulation, and signal stability. Temperature regulation, digestion, physical response, and ordinary movement all require ongoing communication across tissues. Energy is not only inside the system as potential. It must be expressed through the system as function.

This is why energy can be present in the system but poorly expressed through the body. The person may not experience this as a clean mechanical failure. They may experience it as heaviness, reduced ease, faster fatigue, lower tolerance, or difficulty sustaining ordinary output. The felt problem may sound like low energy, even when the limiting layer is not fuel absence.

Communication is therefore an energy requirement. Signals must travel. Nerves must communicate. Muscles must receive instructions. Circulation must deliver fuel, oxygen, fluid, and signaling materials. The body must coordinate many small outputs continuously, not only during deliberate exertion but during ordinary living.

Physical ease depends on communication staying stable under demand. If signals become harder to sustain, ordinary output may feel more effortful. The system may still function, but the cost of function rises. Movement feels less smooth. Posture feels less automatic. Effort feels less durable.

Energy cannot remain usable when the communication layer becomes unstable. The body does not only need material to work with. It needs the conditions that allow instructions, delivery, and response to remain coordinated. Electrolytes matter because they support this signaling environment.

Electrolytes are signal-support infrastructure. In plain terms, they help support electrical signaling, fluid balance, nerve activity, muscle contraction and relaxation, and the gradients that allow signals to move. They are part of the background conditions that make communication possible.

Their role is not to create energy. Their role is to support coordination. This distinction is central. Fuel can supply material. Conversion can turn material into usable work. Electrolyte and fluid balance help the body express that work through signaling, delivery, and physical response.

This is why electrolytes belong in Energy Stability without turning the chapter into a repeat of Electrolytes. The earlier book treats electrolytes as a full system of fluid balance, signaling, and physiological stability. Here, the focus is narrower: how that infrastructure shapes felt energy, fatigue perception, and continuity under demand.

Electrolytes support the signal environment that energy output depends on. When that environment is stable enough, it may go unnoticed. When it becomes strained, the system may feel less coordinated, less tolerant, or less physically easy.

Fluid balance is the circulation side of this same infrastructure. Fluid distribution affects circulation, blood volume, pressure tolerance, delivery, and physical ease. Circulation supports delivery of fuel, oxygen, hormones, and signals. It also supports removal and redistribution. Energy expression depends on this movement.

Pressure tolerance matters because daily function is not performed from one fixed physical state. Standing, changing position, heat exposure, exertion, and ordinary activity all require the system to maintain delivery while conditions change. Poor fluid stability may make these ordinary shifts feel more costly. The person may experience this as heaviness, reduced ease, dizziness, or lower tolerance.

Delivery and tolerance matter for energy continuity. A system that struggles to maintain circulation under ordinary demand may experience energy as unstable even when fuel exists. The issue is not only what is available. It is whether delivery conditions can hold while the body is being used.

Fluid balance supports the delivery conditions that energy continuity depends on.

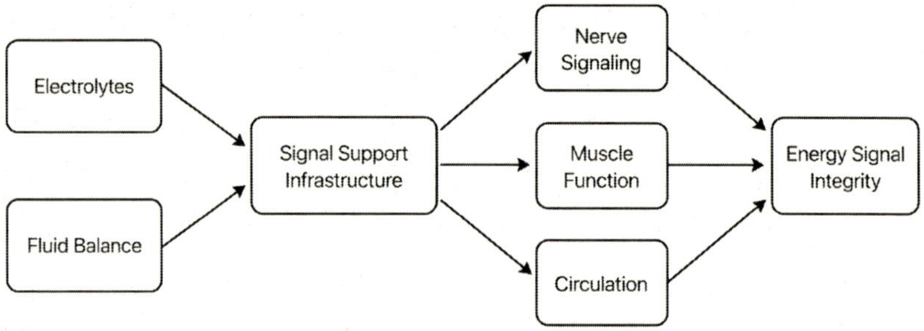

[Figure 16 — Electrolytes and Signal Integrity]

Nerve signaling and muscle function make this infrastructure visible. Energy is felt partly through the ability to move, hold posture, coordinate effort, and sustain physical output. Nerve signals help coordinate action. Muscles require signals to contract and relax. Sustained effort requires repeated signaling, not one signal.

Poor signal support can make effort feel heavy or poorly coordinated. The system may still be able to move, but movement requires more effort. A posture that would normally be held without much awareness may feel costly. A task that is usually automatic may feel less smooth.

Reduced signal integrity can narrow tolerance for ordinary movement. The person may experience this as low energy, but the mechanism may involve signal support rather than fuel supply alone. The body may not be missing all energy; it may be struggling to express energy with ease.

Electrolytes support function; they are not stimulants. They do not create a state of alertness. They help maintain the conditions under which nerve and muscle activity can remain coordinated. Signal integrity affects how usable physical energy feels.

Fatigue perception is the center of this chapter because fatigue is not only lack of fuel. Fatigue can reflect difficulty sustaining coordinated output. When signals, circulation, fluid stability, and muscle response are less supported, the body may interpret the reduced quality of output as fatigue.

Heaviness may reflect higher effort to maintain posture, movement, or circulation. Weakness may reflect difficulty translating signal into action. Dizziness or poor tolerance may reflect circulation or fluid instability. Poor physical ease may reflect signals and delivery not holding smoothly under demand.

This does not mean electrolytes are the cause of all fatigue. Fatigue is a broad signal. It can emerge from sleep constraint, stress load, illness, glucose volatility, under-recovery, transition strain, compensation, or many other layers. The point here is that poor signal support can be experienced as unstable energy.

The body often experiences reduced output quality as a general signal rather than a precise explanation. It does not necessarily announce, in clear language, that fluid distribution is strained or signaling support is less stable. It may simply produce the felt state of heaviness, weakness, reduced tolerance, or faster drop-off.

Poor signal support can be experienced as unstable energy because energy is felt through coordinated output. When coordination becomes costly, output feels less available. This is a mechanism of fatigue perception, not a diagnosis and not a universal explanation.

Electrolytes are a constraint, not a shortcut. They support function, but they do not create fuel. They do not replace sleep, recovery, fuel access, glucose regulation, insulin routing, stress tolerance, transition stability, or conversion capacity. They are one support layer within a larger system.

More is not automatically better. The point of this chapter is not supplementation. The mechanism is about constraints. When electrolyte and fluid support are inadequate, energy expression may become harder. When support is adequate, one constraint is reduced, but that does not guarantee high energy.

This prevents the chapter from becoming an electrolyte solution chapter. Energy stability is not achieved by turning one infrastructure layer into the whole explanation. Electrolytes matter because the system needs signal integrity and fluid stability. They do not become the system itself.

Electrolytes are infrastructure, not an energy source. Their importance is indirect but essential. They support the conditions through which energy becomes usable, physical, coordinated, and durable under ordinary demand.

Electrolyte and fluid balance also exist in system context. Fasting and meal timing can change fluid and electrolyte dynamics. Sweating and heat can increase fluid and electrolyte demand. Illness can disrupt fluid stability. Stress can alter tension, fluid perception, and tolerance. Sleep and recovery affect regulatory stability. Activity changes circulation, muscle use, and fluid needs.

The same electrolyte or fluid state may feel different under different conditions. After poor sleep, signal tolerance may be lower. Under stress load, physical tension and readiness demand may increase cost. In heat or during activity, circulation and fluid distribution may be more heavily tested. During illness, the system may allocate resources differently.

Electrolyte meaning depends on the surrounding system state. It should not be isolated from demand load, recovery, stress, sleep, activity, appetite, glucose, or fuel transitions. The felt effect of this layer depends on what the rest of the system is asking it to support.

Energy continuity requires signal support that holds under demand. Ordinary demand is not static. Standing, walking, working, digesting, regulating temperature, and responding to stress all require ongoing coordination. Tolerance means the system can sustain output without signals degrading quickly.

When electrolyte or fluid strain reduces tolerance, energy may drop off faster. Physical ease may decline. Effort may become less smooth. The system may need more compensation to maintain output. This connects directly to the Energy Continuity Mechanism because stable energy is not only output at one moment; it is output sustained across time without excessive disruption.

Poor signal support can look like low energy even when fuel is present. Fuel may be available. Conversion may be possible. But signals may be poorly supported. Circulation may feel strained. Movement may feel harder. Posture may feel less durable. Physical ease may decline.

The body may interpret poor coordination as fatigue. This does not mean the person lacks energy in a simple inventory sense. It means energy expression is constrained. The usable output is reduced because the communication and delivery layer is under strain.

Energy can feel low when signal support is weak, even if fuel exists. This completes the chain from fuel availability to conversion to expression. Fuel must become reachable. Reachable fuel must become usable. Usable energy must still be expressed through coordinated physical systems.

Electrolytes are one constraint layer, not the whole system. Electrolyte and fluid balance matter because signal integrity matters. But energy also depends on glucose, insulin, appetite, sleep, stress, recovery, fuel access, conversion, transition tolerance, and demand load. Identical electrolyte conditions may feel different under different sleep, stress, heat, activity, illness, or fasting states.

This layer should be interpreted in context, not isolated. It matters because the body needs communication and circulation to express energy. It does not matter because electrolytes are the whole answer.

The Electrolyte Constraint Mechanism explains how electrolyte and fluid balance affect energy continuity by supporting signal transmission, circulation, nerve activity, muscle function, fluid distribution, pressure tolerance, and fatigue perception. It includes communication, circulation, fluid balance, pressure tolerance, signal transmission, nerve activity, muscle contraction, muscle relaxation, cellular gradients, physical ease, heaviness, dizziness, weakness, fatigue perception, tolerance under demand, system context, and continuity impact.

Electrolytes do not create energy. They support the signaling and fluid conditions that allow energy to be expressed. Their role is infrastructural, and their meaning depends on the demands placed on the system around them.

Electrolyte and fluid balance show how physical signal support can shape fatigue perception and energy continuity. But by this point in the book, energy instability has been shown across multiple layers: fuel access, conversion, transitions, crashes, drift, compensation, glucose, insulin, appetite, sleep, stress, and signal support. The next step is learning how to recognize patterns without reducing them to one cause. The next chapter turns to the Pattern Recognition Mechanism.

Pattern Recognition Mechanism

Identifying stable versus unstable energy patterns.

Energy fluctuations are easy to overinterpret because they are felt directly. A dip can feel like failure. A strong morning can feel like proof that the system is stable. A crash can seem random because the decline is experienced more clearly than the conditions that built it. Without pattern recognition, energy becomes a collection of isolated moments, each one interpreted too quickly.

A single moment rarely explains the system. One low period does not define energy stability. One strong day does not prove full continuity. One crash does not identify one cause. Energy is a time-based output, and time-based outputs cannot be understood by isolating one reading, one sensation, or one episode from the larger pattern.

The goal is not to micromanage every energy fluctuation; the goal is to recognize recurring patterns across time.

Energy stability becomes interpretable when its shape is visible. One moment shows output, but pattern requires timing, recurrence, recovery, disruption, and trajectory. The same dip has different meaning depending on whether it appears once after unusual demand or repeatedly after ordinary demand. The same fatigue has different meaning depending on whether recovery returns quickly or remains delayed.

Timing matters because energy changes across the day. Morning energy, post-meal energy, afternoon energy, evening fatigue, post-stress fatigue, and next-day recovery are not interchangeable signals. A dip after poor sleep carries a different meaning from a dip after a meal, activity, stress, or long demand period. Energy becomes more readable when the timing of change is placed beside the conditions surrounding it.

Recovery matters because stable systems move and return. A fluctuation that resolves without major disruption carries a different meaning from one that requires compensation, narrows function, or leaves the next period weaker. Disruption matters because not every change interrupts life. Trajectory matters because baseline can remain steady, gradually lower, or become less predictable.

Normal rhythm is not instability. Stable energy is not perfectly flat energy. Biological systems move. Energy varies with time of day, meals, activity, sleep, demand, recovery, stress load, appetite signals, glucose movement, and transition state. A stable pattern may include dips, lower-output windows, hunger, and fatigue toward the end of the day.

The question is not whether energy changes. The question is whether those changes remain proportionate, recoverable, and integrated into continuity. A mild dip that fits the context and resolves without major strain is different from a repeated sharp drop that interrupts function. Rhythm allows movement. Instability disrupts continuity.

Stable energy allows rhythm; unstable energy disrupts continuity. This distinction protects the reader from flat-energy thinking. A stable system can rise, soften, recover, and shift without becoming unstable. The stability is in the continuity, not in sameness.

Stable patterns tend to be smoother, recoverable, proportionate, and less disruptive. Smooth does not mean flat. It means transitions are not abrupt enough to break function repeatedly. Recoverable means the system returns to usable output without major compensation. Proportionate means the energy change fits the demand or context. Less disruptive means function remains broadly intact even as energy moves.

Stable patterns often have recognizable rhythm rather than chaotic swings. The person may feel more alert at one time, softer at another, lower after demand, and restored after recovery. These changes do not require constant interpretation. They fit the system's ordinary movement.

Stable patterns preserve function even when energy moves. They do not require the person to manage every shift, explain every sensation, or treat every dip as a problem. They allow ordinary variability while maintaining usable output across time.

Unstable patterns are different. They tend to be recurrent, sharp, delayed, compensatory, or progressively worsening. Recurrent means the same kind of disruption repeats in a recognizable way. Sharp means the change is abrupt or disproportionate to the visible context. Delayed means the cost appears after the cause is less visible. Compensatory means output depends on activation or short-term supports. Progressively worsening means baseline, recovery, or tolerance is deteriorating.

An unstable pattern disrupts continuity rather than merely changing energy. It may force repeated recovery, narrow the day's range, increase urgency, create crashes, require compensation, or make ordinary demand feel increasingly costly. The instability is not in the existence of movement. It is in the pattern's recurrence, shape, cost, and effect on function.

Unstable patterns reveal themselves through recurrence, sharpness, delay, compensation, or worsening trajectory.

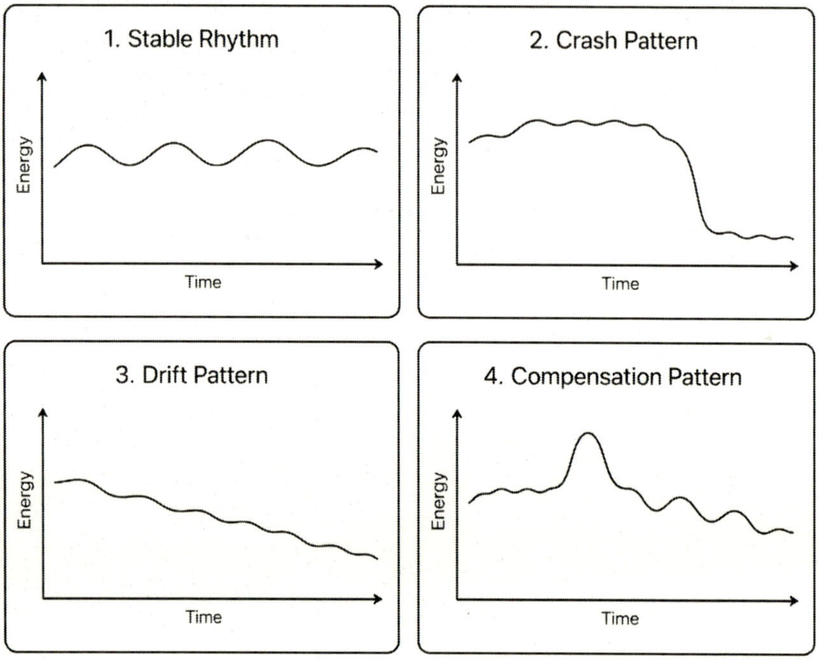

[Figure 17 — Energy Pattern Recognition]

A crash pattern is a rapid loss of usable output after temporary elevation or apparent stability. It is sharper than an ordinary dip. Energy may appear available, output may be holding, and then function drops quickly. The decline may feel sudden, but the chain often began earlier.

Crash patterns may appear after activation, glucose volatility, poor sleep, stress load, transition strain, or compensation. The system may have been functioning through temporary support before output fell. This is why the crash should not be interpreted only at the moment of decline. The pattern includes what preceded it.

A crash pattern is a rapid loss of usable output after the system appeared to be functioning. Recurrence matters because one crash may reflect a specific context, while repeated crashes suggest a continuity pattern that deserves broader interpretation.

A drift pattern is slower. Drift is gradual downward movement in baseline energy. It may become familiar before it becomes obvious. Instead of a sharp drop, the system begins operating from a lower starting point. Tasks require more effort. Recovery takes longer. Activity tolerance narrows. Compensation becomes more common.

Drift is not one tired day. A single low day may reflect sleep, stress, illness, demand, or context. Drift becomes clearer when the baseline itself appears to be moving. The person may adjust expectations, reduce range, or treat lower output as normal because the change occurred gradually.

A drift pattern is baseline lowering across time, not one isolated low day. Recurrence matters because drift is visible through trajectory, not through a single episode.

A compensation cycle pattern occurs when short-term supports repeatedly preserve function under unstable conditions. Compensation may look like strength from the outside because output continues. The person may still complete tasks, maintain routines, respond to demand, or appear functional. But the output may be supported by activation, urgency, habit, external demand, narrowed routines, or forced continuation.

Compensation is not the same as resilience. Resilience implies recovery and restored capacity. Compensation may preserve function without restoring the underlying system. The cost may appear later as fatigue, appetite disruption, sleep disruption, irritability, crash, or drift.

A compensation cycle is repeated short-term function that increases future instability cost. Recurrence matters because compensation becomes more destabilizing when it becomes the default operating mode rather than a temporary bridge.

An overactivation pattern appears when readiness stays elevated beyond the immediate need. The system may feel alert, urgent, restless, unable to settle, or driven by pressure rather than restored capacity. Output may be present, but it may not be durable.

Overactivation is different from stable energy because fatigue can coexist with activation. A person may feel wired and depleted at the same time. Sleep, appetite, glucose, stress signals, and recovery may become less stable because the system remains oriented toward response.

An overactivation pattern is energy that feels available because readiness remains elevated, not because capacity is restored. Recurrence matters because repeated overactivation can increase compensation pressure, reduce recovery bandwidth, and contribute to volatility.

Post-meal dips require careful interpretation. A post-meal dip is not automatically one cause. It may involve glucose variability, insulin routing, digestion cost, sleep debt, stress state, appetite and satiety mismatch, prior demand, recovery state, or transition tolerance. The meal matters, but the system receiving the meal also matters.

Pattern matters more than one episode. Timing, severity, recurrence, and recovery determine whether the post-meal dip is an isolated response or a repeated instability pattern. A mild softening after eating is not the same as a recurrent, disruptive drop that appears consistently and takes significant recovery.

A post-meal dip becomes meaningful when its timing, recurrence, severity, and recovery pattern are consistent. This prevents the pattern from being reduced to a single food, a single glucose explanation, or a moral interpretation of eating.

Delayed fatigue appears after demand rather than during it. The system may perform during the task, social period, activity, stressor, or long day, then pay later. The cost may appear hours later, in the evening, the next morning, or after the activating condition has passed.

Delayed fatigue reveals hidden cost. It shows that output can be possible without being durable. Sleep constraint, stress load, compensation, activity demand, transition strain, and reduced recovery capacity can all contribute. The key feature is timing: the fatigue appears after the output rather than interrupting it immediately.

Delayed fatigue shows that the cost of output may appear after the output itself. Recurrence matters because repeated delayed fatigue suggests that visible function is being maintained at a cost the system cannot fully absorb.

Load mismatch prepares the next mechanism. Load mismatch occurs when demand repeatedly exceeds available capacity. The same demand can produce different energy outcomes depending on system state. A task that is tolerable after good restoration may be destabilizing after poor sleep. A meal, walk, workday, stressor, or fasting interval may feel different depending on baseline, recovery, fuel access, transition tolerance, and signal support.

Load includes physical, cognitive, emotional, metabolic, environmental, and recovery load. Capacity includes sleep, recovery, fuel access, conversion, stress tolerance, electrolyte and fluid support, transition stability, and baseline energy. When load exceeds capacity, the system may show faster fatigue, sharper dips, compensation, poor recovery, or next-day decline.

A load mismatch pattern appears when demand repeatedly exceeds the system's available capacity. Recurrence matters because mismatch is relational. It is not only the demand and not only the person's energy state. It is the comparison between the two across time.

Isolated episodes must be treated carefully. One bad day is not automatically a pattern. One strong day is not automatically stability. One crash does not explain the whole system. A pattern requires recurrence, timing, recovery, disruption, and trajectory.

This prevents overreaction. If every fluctuation is treated as meaningful, interpretation becomes unstable. The reader begins responding to moments instead of patterns. A single dip becomes a problem to solve. A single strong morning becomes proof that the system has fully recovered. A single crash becomes a complete explanation.

Pattern recognition also prevents underreaction. Repeated signals matter. A recurring crash, worsening baseline, delayed fatigue pattern, or repeated compensation cycle should not be dismissed simply because each individual episode can be explained away. Pattern recognition holds both truths together: isolated episodes can be misleading, and repeated patterns carry information.

Pattern recognition prevents both overreaction to isolated episodes and underreaction to recurring instability.

The Pattern Recognition Mechanism explains how energy stability is interpreted by reading energy across time, distinguishing normal rhythm from recurrent instability, and identifying whether changes appear as crashes, drift, overactivation, delayed fatigue, post-meal dips, compensation cycles, or load mismatch. It includes rhythm, recurrence, timing, severity, recovery, disruption, delay, compensation, trajectory, baseline movement, load context, system state, and continuity impact.

The goal is not to micromanage every energy fluctuation. The goal is to recognize recurring patterns across time. Energy is a system output, and system outputs become meaningful when their shape, timing, cost, and recovery are seen together.

Pattern recognition shows what is happening across time. The next question is why the pattern appears under some conditions and not others. That requires comparing load against capacity. A demand that is tolerable under one system state may become destabilizing under another. The next chapter turns to the Load vs Capacity Mechanism.

Load vs Capacity Mechanism

Mismatch between demand and recovery.

Energy instability is often interpreted as a problem with one visible demand. The workout was too much. The meal caused the dip. The workday was too long. The night of sleep was poor. The stressful event was the cause. The fasting window was the problem. The schedule was too busy. These visible demands attract attention because they are easy to identify. They appear close to the energy change, so they seem to explain it.

That interpretation is understandable, but incomplete. A visible demand rarely arrives alone. It arrives into a system already shaped by prior sleep, recovery state, stress load, fuel access, appetite pressure, glucose movement, transition tolerance, signal support, and baseline energy. The same demand can be absorbed in one state and destabilizing in another.

Energy instability is often not caused by one demand alone, but by repeated mismatch between total load and available capacity.

Load is the total demand placed on the system. It is broader than exercise, work, or stress. Physical activity is load because movement requires fuel, circulation, signal coordination, muscle function, and recovery. Work demand is load because attention, decision-making, communication, and sustained focus consume regulatory capacity. Cognitive demand is load because thinking, planning, filtering, and responding require energy continuity even when the body is physically still.

Emotional demand is also load. Conflict, uncertainty, caregiving, pressure, responsibility, and anticipation all create readiness costs. Stress is load because it redirects the system toward response. Illness is load because immune activity and recovery needs change resource allocation. Heat, environmental pressure, schedule instability, social demand, and decision load all add to what the system must carry.

Metabolic transitions are load as well. Feeding, fasting, glucose movement, fuel switching, appetite pressure, digestion, and transition states all require coordination. These are not failures. They are ordinary processes. But they still place demands on the system.

Poor sleep and recovery debt increase load because they make ordinary demand more expensive. The same task requires more from a less-restored system. The same meal may feel different. The same stressor may feel sharper. The same activity may produce more recovery cost. Load is not one event; it is the total demand the system must carry.

Capacity is the system's ability to absorb demand while maintaining usable output and returning toward recovery. It includes sleep quality, recovery state, fuel access, conversion capacity, transition tolerance, stress tolerance, movement tolerance, glucose stability, insulin coordination, appetite stability, electrolyte and fluid support, signal stability, recovery bandwidth, and baseline energy.

Capacity is not fixed. It changes with prior conditions. A system beginning the day with better restoration, smoother fuel access, lower stress activation, and stronger signal support has more room to absorb demand. A system beginning with poor sleep, accumulated strain, appetite disruption, glucose volatility, or stress load has less margin.

Capacity is therefore not motivation or willingness. It is the available ability to absorb load without losing continuity. When capacity is higher, ordinary demands may pass through the system with less disruption. When capacity is lower, the same demands may produce fatigue, volatility, compensation, or delayed cost.

The relationship between load and capacity matters more than either side alone. High load does not automatically create instability if capacity is sufficient. A demanding day may be absorbed when restoration, fuel access, stress tolerance, and recovery bandwidth are strong enough. A lower or ordinary load can become destabilizing when capacity is reduced.

This explains why energy can feel inconsistent without requiring moral judgment. A demand that is tolerable one day may be destabilizing another day. The difference is not necessarily character, discipline, or effort. It may be the relationship between the demand and the capacity available to absorb it.

Energy outcome depends on the relationship between load and capacity.

When load stays within capacity, output can continue with less disruption. The system may still use energy, shift state, and require recovery, but continuity remains intact. Variation may occur, but it remains proportionate and recoverable.

When load approaches capacity, effort rises. Recovery need increases. Signals may become more noticeable. Hunger, fatigue, irritability, heaviness, or urgency may begin to appear. The system is still functioning, but the margin is narrowing.

When load exceeds capacity, fatigue, volatility, compensation, or instability appears. This crossing can happen sharply, as in a crash, or gradually, as in drift. It can happen after one unusually demanding event, but repeated crossings matter more because they change future capacity.

The system may still function above capacity temporarily. Output can continue through activation, urgency, routine, social demand, narrowed options, or forced continuation. But continued output does not mean the load was absorbable. It may mean the cost has been deferred.

Load crossing capacity triggers fatigue, compensation, and instability.

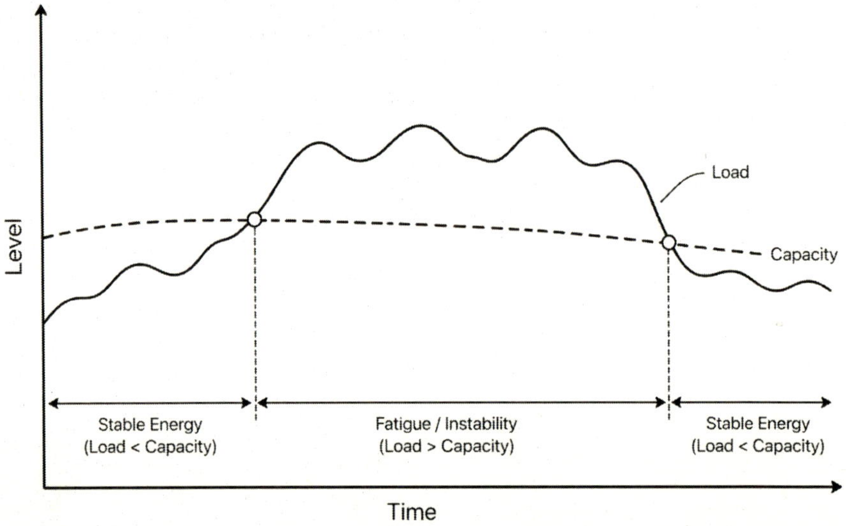

[Figure 18 — Load vs Capacity]

Temporary function above capacity is compensation. A person may continue working, moving, responding, deciding, or meeting obligations even when the system's absorbable capacity has been exceeded. Output continues because support systems are recruited: activation, urgency, routine, narrowed output, external demand, or forced continuation.

This can make mismatch difficult to see. From the outside, the person may appear functional. From the inside, output may feel effortful, brittle, or dependent on pressure. The day may be completed, but the system may have accumulated cost.

Temporary function above capacity is compensation, not proof that load was tolerable. This distinction matters because compensation can hide mismatch until later. Energy continuity may be strained even while output is still present.

Repeated mismatch can produce fatigue because output has repeatedly exceeded absorbable demand. The fatigue may not appear immediately. It may appear after repeated ordinary demands, after several days of reduced restoration, after chronic stress activation, or after a period of functioning through compensation.

This fatigue can feel disproportionate because the visible demand was only part of the total load. The person may look at the most recent task and wonder why it produced such a strong effect. But the task may have landed on top of poor sleep, stress load, appetite pressure, glucose volatility, illness load, or recovery debt.

Fatigue can reflect accumulated mismatch, not only the most recent demand. This is why delayed fatigue can be confusing. The system may perform during demand and show the cost later, when the original load is no longer visible.

Repeated mismatch can also make crashes more likely. The system may hold output temporarily through activation or compensation. Energy may appear stable for a time. Then, when compensatory support can no longer maintain output, function drops sharply.

A crash may follow stress activation, glucose volatility, poor sleep, transition strain, high demand, or irregular recovery. It may appear sudden because the decline is felt suddenly, but the mismatch may have been building earlier. Load may have exceeded capacity before the crash was visible.

A crash can occur when load has been carried beyond capacity until output can no longer be held.

Repeated mismatch can also lower baseline over time. If recovery does not restore prior capacity, the next period begins lower. The system starts with less margin. Ordinary load becomes more costly. Compensation becomes more common. Recovery becomes less complete.

This is drift. It is not a sharp failure. It is a gradual lowering of the starting point. The system continues, but from a reduced baseline. Each repeated mismatch makes the next load harder to absorb.

Drift can emerge when repeated mismatch lowers the starting point for future energy.

Mismatch also affects the signals that help determine future capacity. Load beyond capacity can alter appetite pressure. Hunger may become stronger, delayed, or more urgent. Satiety may become less durable. Cravings may narrow attention around fast resolution.

Glucose movement may feel more volatile under mismatch because the system is carrying more demand with less margin. The same glucose pattern may feel different under poor sleep, stress load, or recovery debt. Sleep may become less restorative when stress activation or compensatory output remains high. Stress activation may increase as the system tries to maintain output.

These secondary effects can feed into future load and capacity. Appetite disruption, sleep disruption, glucose volatility, and stress activation do not remain isolated. They shape the next cycle of energy continuity. Mismatch can disturb the signals that help determine future capacity.

The same load can produce different outcomes depending on available capacity. A workload may feel tolerable after better sleep and destabilizing after poor restoration. A meal may feel steady in one context and heavy in another. An activity may feel manageable when recovery is adequate and costly when recovery debt is present. A fasting interval, social event, or stressor may feel different depending on baseline state.

Under stress, capacity may be lower because readiness demand is already high. During illness, capacity may be redirected toward recovery. In heat, circulation and fluid support may be more heavily tested. During transition strain, fuel access and conversion may require more coordination. Under recovery debt, ordinary demand may exceed capacity more quickly.

This explains why energy outcomes vary without requiring moral judgment. The same load can be stable or destabilizing depending on available capacity.

Load-capacity mismatch is not laziness, weakness, or a character problem. It describes a relationship between demand and the system's ability to absorb demand. A system can be overloaded by cumulative demand even when each individual demand is ordinary.

This protects interpretation from two errors. The first is self-blame, where every fatigue signal becomes a personal failure. The second is oversimplification, where one visible demand is treated as the entire cause. Both miss the relational nature of energy stability.

Mismatch describes a relationship between demand and capacity, not a judgment about the person.

The Load vs Capacity Mechanism explains how energy instability emerges when total demand repeatedly exceeds the system's available capacity to absorb, regulate, recover, and sustain output. It includes load, capacity, cumulative demand, recovery state, sleep quality, fuel access, conversion capacity, transition tolerance, stress tolerance, movement tolerance, signal stability, appetite stability, glucose stability, electrolyte and fluid support, compensation, fatigue, crashes, baseline drift, secondary signal disruption, and continuity impact.

Energy instability is often not caused by one demand alone, but by repeated mismatch between total load and available capacity. This model integrates the book's prior mechanisms into one relationship: what the system must carry, and what the system can absorb.

Load versus capacity gives the reader the simplest integrative model in the book. Energy remains more stable when demand stays within absorbable capacity and becomes less stable when demand repeatedly exceeds it. The final chapter turns from interpretation to stability framing, integrating fuel, signals, recovery, constraints, patterns, load, and capacity into a complete model of energy as system output.

Stability Framing Mechanism

Energy as a system output, not a target.

Energy is often treated as something to increase directly. When it is high, it is read as success. When it drops, it is read as failure. When it feels absent, the first impulse is often to recover it quickly, force it upward, or identify the single factor that removed it. This is understandable because energy is felt immediately. It is not abstract. It appears in the body as readiness, heaviness, clarity, fog, movement, fatigue, urgency, or resistance.

Because energy is so immediate, it is easy to mistake the felt state for the whole system. A strong day can seem to prove that the system is working well. A low day can seem to prove that something has failed. A crash can feel like a sudden defect. A period of high output can feel like stability because output is visible. But energy is not the system itself. It is the real-time functional expression of the system beneath it.

Energy stability is continuity, not intensity.

This distinction has carried the entire book. Energy is not best understood as a fixed resource, motivational state, productivity tool, personality trait, or peak-performance target. It is not discipline. It is not stimulation. It is not proof of virtue. It is not a moral signal. Energy is a system output, and outputs must be interpreted before they are targeted.

When energy is treated as something to force, the system underneath can be missed. A person may focus on the feeling of low energy without seeing the load that preceded it. They may focus on a temporary high without seeing the compensation carrying it. They may focus on one meal, one night of sleep, one stressful period, or one crash, while the broader pattern remains unseen. Direct targeting narrows attention to the surface.

Continuity is the proper measure because energy stability is not defined by how high output rises. It is defined by whether usable output can hold across time without excessive peaks, crashes, drift, or compensatory strain. A system can produce a high-energy window and still be unstable if that window is followed by collapse, prolonged recovery, or increasing dependence on activation.

Continuity does not mean flat energy. A living system moves. Energy rises with demand, softens during recovery, changes after meals, shifts with sleep state, responds to stress, and varies across the day. Stability allows rhythm. It allows lower-output periods. It allows fatigue when demand has accumulated. It allows recovery windows. Flatness is not the standard.

Stable energy is energy that remains usable, recoverable, and less disruptive across time. The question is not whether energy changes. The question is whether those changes preserve function, return proportionately, and avoid repeated strain. Continuity is not sameness. It is the durable coherence of output under ordinary conditions.

The system beneath energy is layered. Fuel must be accessible, not merely present. Food entering the body, stored reserves, or circulating fuel do not automatically become stable daily energy. Fuel must be mobilized, transported, coordinated, and matched to demand. Availability matters because energy cannot be sustained if fuel cannot reach the places where function requires it.

Accessible fuel must also be converted. Available fuel is not the same as usable energy. Conversion depends on cellular uptake, oxygen delivery, circulation, mitochondrial function, current demand, recovery state, stress load, and conversion tolerance. Fuel may be present and reachable while output still feels strained if the system cannot convert it smoothly under current conditions.

Transitions must be tolerated. The body does not remain in one fuel state all day. It shifts between fed and fasting conditions, more glucose-dominant and more fat-dominant reliance, rest and activity, demand and recovery. Energy can become unstable not because one state is inherently wrong, but because movement between states is poorly tolerated. Transition stability supports continuity.

Glucose matters, but it is not the whole system. Glucose patterns can influence alertness, urgency, dips, hunger, fog, post-meal energy, and crash risk. But glucose movement must be interpreted in context: insulin signaling, sleep, stress, appetite, recovery, activity, transition tolerance, and demand load all shape how glucose is handled and felt.

Insulin also belongs in context. It is not good or bad. It is a routing signal that shapes energy distribution and access. It helps determine whether fuel remains circulating, moves into use, enters storage, or becomes less accessible under current conditions. Storage is not failure. Routing is not blame. Energy continuity depends on whether routing, demand, access, and recovery remain coordinated.

Appetite becomes the behavioral interface of the energy system. Hunger, cravings, muted appetite, and satiety loss are connected to energy, but they are not identical to energy. Appetite may forecast need, reflect perceived availability, respond to glucose and insulin patterns, shift under stress, change after poor sleep, or become distorted by compensation. Appetite signals influence future energy because they shape eating response, but they do not perfectly reveal current energy state.

Sleep restores the system that energy must come from. It is not merely rest. It shapes next-day baseline, glucose handling, appetite pressure, stress tolerance, recovery capacity, nervous system readiness, rhythm, and metabolic regulation. Poor restoration can lower baseline and increase volatility. The same demand can feel different depending on the recovery state that receives it.

Stress redirects readiness and increases cost. Temporary activation may raise alertness, urgency, and output, but activation is not durable capacity. A person can feel wired and depleted at the same time because readiness and restoration are different layers. Stress load can preserve function briefly while reducing recovery bandwidth and increasing future volatility.

Electrolytes and fluid balance support the physical expression of energy. They do not create energy. They support signal transmission, circulation, pressure tolerance, nerve activity, muscle function, and fatigue perception. Energy must be expressed through the body. Fuel and conversion are not enough if signals, delivery, and physical coordination are strained.

Recovery bandwidth determines whether the system can restore after demand. Load and capacity determine whether continuity holds. Energy becomes more stable when the systems beneath it hold together with less volatility.

Fatigue belongs inside this frame. Fatigue is not weakness, laziness, lack of character, or failure. It is a signal that usable output is becoming constrained. It can reflect fuel access, conversion strain, sleep limitation, stress load, recovery debt, glucose volatility, appetite misalignment, electrolyte and fluid strain, compensation, illness load, or demand exceeding capacity.

Fatigue may be immediate or delayed. It may appear during demand, after demand, later in the day, or the next morning. It may be felt as heaviness, fog, reduced tolerance, slower recovery, irritability, or loss of momentum. The sensation is real, but it is not self-explanatory. It requires context.

This does not mean fatigue should be dismissed or explained away. It means fatigue should not be moralized. Fatigue is information about the system. It signals that continuity is being strained, that recovery may be incomplete, that output may be exceeding capacity, or that some layer beneath energy is not holding smoothly.

Crashes and drift also belong to pattern interpretation. A crash is rapid output loss after temporary elevation, apparent stability, or compensatory activation. It feels sudden, but it is often built before it appears. The visible drop may be the endpoint of earlier strain.

Drift is slower. It is gradual baseline lowering over time. It may become familiar before it becomes obvious. The system does not collapse sharply; it begins operating from a lower starting point. Ordinary demand feels more expensive. Recovery becomes less complete. Compensation becomes more common.

Both crashes and drift become meaningful when read as patterns across time. A single crash does not define the system. One tired day is not drift. But recurrence, timing, recovery cost, and trajectory reveal whether instability is forming. Pattern recognition protects against both overreaction and dismissal.

Compensation explains why instability can remain hidden. A person can continue functioning while the system becomes less stable. Output may be preserved through activation, urgency, narrowed routines, external demand, habit, stimulation, or forced continuation. From the outside, function may look intact. From the system's perspective, continuity may be maintained at higher cost.

Compensation is not failure. It is a short-term preservation strategy. Life often requires temporary supports. The issue is not that compensation exists. The issue is whether compensation becomes a substitute for restoration. Temporary function does not prove durable capacity.

Compensation can maintain output temporarily without restoring the system beneath it. This is why high output is not always evidence of stability. A system may continue until cost appears later as fatigue, appetite disruption, sleep disruption, irritability, crash, drift, or lower tolerance.

Load and capacity provide the simplest integrative model. Load is total demand. Capacity is the available ability to absorb demand while maintaining usable output and returning toward recovery. Energy continuity holds when demand remains within absorbable capacity. Instability emerges when load repeatedly exceeds capacity.

Load includes physical activity, cognitive demand, work demand, emotional demand, stress, illness, heat, social demand, decision load, schedule instability, metabolic transitions, glucose movement, appetite pressure, poor sleep, and recovery debt. Capacity includes sleep quality, recovery state, fuel access, conversion tolerance, stress tolerance, movement tolerance, glucose stability, insulin coordination, appetite stability, electrolyte and fluid support, signal integrity, baseline energy, and recovery bandwidth.

The same demand can be stable or destabilizing depending on state. A meal, workday, activity, social event, fasting interval, or stressor does not have the same effect in every context. Demand arrives into a system with a current capacity. That capacity changes.

Energy continuity depends on the relationship between total load and available capacity. This relationship integrates sleep, stress, fuel, appetite, recovery, glucose, insulin, electrolytes, movement, and environmental demand into one frame. Energy instability is often not caused by one demand alone, but by repeated mismatch between what the system must carry and what it can absorb.

This is why energy should not be chased directly. Chasing energy focuses on the felt output while often missing the conditions producing it. Forcing output can increase compensation. Treating every dip as a target can create overreaction. Treating every high as stability can hide drift. Treating every crash as random can miss the chain that built it.

Energy is feedback from the system, not a separate object to force. It gives information about continuity, recovery, load, capacity, signal coordination, and constraint. The felt state matters, but it is not the whole explanation. Energy is real, but it is produced.

The Stability Framing Mechanism explains how energy should be interpreted as a real-time functional output of metabolic stability rather than a direct target to chase, force, maximize, or moralize. It includes continuity, rhythm, fuel access, conversion, transitions, glucose, insulin, appetite, sleep, stress, electrolytes, recovery, crashes, drift, compensation, pattern recognition, load, capacity, fatigue perception, and system output.

Energy becomes more stable when the systems beneath it hold together with less volatility. That is the final frame of the book. Stability is not the pursuit of constant elevation. It is the preservation of usable function across time through coordinated regulation, adequate recovery, tolerable transitions, proportionate load, and reduced compensatory strain.

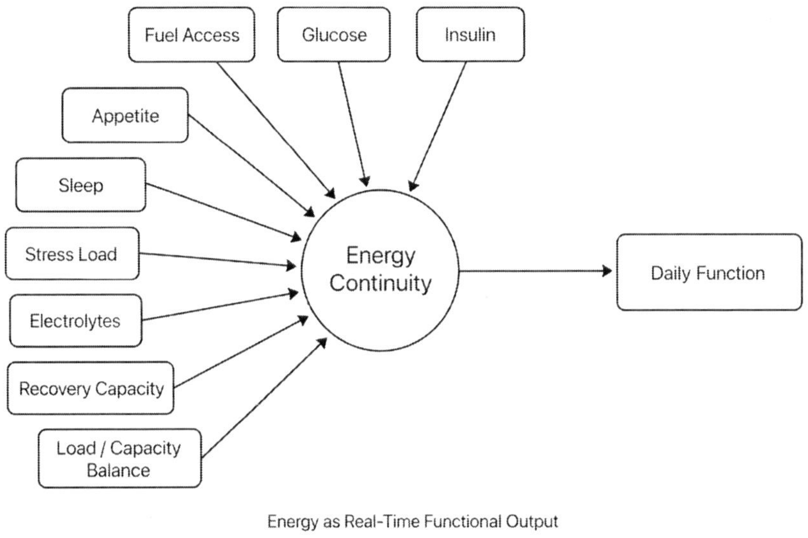

[Figure 19 — Energy Stability Integration Model]

Energy stability is not a promise of constant high energy. It is not a guarantee that fatigue disappears, dips never occur, or output remains identical every hour. It is a way of understanding why energy holds, fluctuates, crashes, drifts, or recovers.

Energy is real. Fatigue is meaningful. Instability has patterns. Crashes and drift are not isolated moral failures. Compensation is not proof of strength or weakness. Appetite, glucose, insulin, sleep, stress, electrolytes, recovery, load, and capacity all shape the conditions from which daily function emerges.

The purpose of this frame is not to turn energy into another target. It is to return energy to its proper place. Energy is the visible and felt expression of whether the system beneath it is holding together across time.

Energy stability is continuity, not intensity. It is the real-time functional output of metabolic stability.

About the Author

Nathan Reed writes about metabolic stability in systems exposed to load, variability, and time.

His work examines how biological capacity is shaped by energy availability, recovery architecture, sleep amplitude, muscle mass, environmental demand and workload. Rather than treating nutrition, fasting, sleep, and training as isolated tactics, he approaches them as interacting regulatory systems governed by margin, buffering, oscillatory coherence, and constraint dominance.

The Stability framework explores how physiological compression accumulates gradually and how proportional calibration preserves long-horizon resilience across decades. The objective is not peak optimization, but preservation of functional continuity under load.

Energy Stability is part of a broader metabolic stability ecosystem developed under Perennial Publishing, each volume addressing a distinct vector of biological durability.

The work is designed for readers who prefer structural clarity over motivational rhetoric and long-horizon coherence over short-term intensity.

The Metabolic Stability Series

Metabolic Stability: *A Systems Guide to Blood Sugar, Fasting, and Long-Term Metabolic Health*

(Cornerstone Volume)

Fasting Fundamentals: *A Systems Guide to Metabolic Flexibility, Fat Loss, and Long-Term Health*

(Foundational Volume)

Intermittent Fasting: *Metabolic Timing, Body Composition, and Sustainable Health*

Prolonged Fasting: *A Systems Guide to Duration, Recovery, and Metabolic Limits*

Electrolytes: *A Systems Guide to Hydration, Electrolyte Balance, and Physiological Stability*

Insulin Stability: *Blood Sugar, Insulin Resistance, and Metabolic Health*

Glucose Stability: *How Blood Sugar Fluctuations Affect Energy, Insulin, and Metabolic Health*

Metabolic Flexibility: *How the Body Switches Between Fat and Glucose for Energy and Metabolic Health*

Appetite Stability: *How Hunger, Satiety, Cravings, and Energy Signals Shape Eating Behavior*

Energy Stability: *How the Body Regulates Fuel, Fatigue, Recovery, and Daily Function*

Future Titles Include:

Fat Loss Stability

The Vitality Series:

Sleep and Recovery

Strength and Aging

Hormones & Sexual Health

Part of a Broader Stability Framework

The Metabolic Stability Series is part of a larger stability ecosystem published by Perennial Publishing.

Related domains include:

Money Stability — structural durability in financial systems

Career Stability — positioning, load tolerance, and transition resilience

Mental Stability — cognitive steadiness under pressure and uncertainty

Emotional Stability — regulatory steadiness in environments that do not slow down

Foundations — low-fragility life architecture

Vitality — energy, strength, and biological function across time

Each domain approaches stability as a structural problem: capacity versus load, buffering versus shock, governance versus drift. Together, they form a unified framework for long-horizon durability across the major systems that shape human trajectory.

About Perennial Publishing

Perennial Publishing produces practical systems guides for building stability in an unstable world.

Our books explore the foundations of long-term resilience across health, finance, career, and everyday decision-making. Each title focuses on clear frameworks, durable principles, and practical strategies that help readers build lasting stability rather than short-term fixes.

The Perennial catalog includes series on metabolic health, financial stability, career systems, and personal consistency. While each book stands on its own, they share a common goal: helping individuals create durable systems that support a stable and sustainable life.